The Trying Time

The Trying Time

A Comprehensive Guide to Infertility, IVF, and Family Building

Jessica Manns

BLOOMSBURY ACADEMIC
NEW YORK • LONDON • OXFORD • NEW DELHI • SYDNEY

BLOOMSBURY ACADEMIC
Bloomsbury Publishing Inc, 1359 Broadway, New York, NY 10018, USA
Bloomsbury Publishing Plc, 50 Bedford Square, London, WC1B 3DP, UK
Bloomsbury Publishing Ireland, 29 Earlsfort Terrace, Dublin 2, D02 AY28, Ireland

BLOOMSBURY, BLOOMSBURY ACADEMIC and the Diana logo are trademarks of
Bloomsbury Publishing Plc

First published in the United States of America 2025

Copyright © Jessica Manns, 2025

Cover image © Jessica Manns

All rights reserved. No part of this publication may be: i) reproduced or transmitted in any form, electronic or mechanical, including photocopying, recording or by means of any information storage or retrieval system without prior permission in writing from the publishers; or ii) used or reproduced in any way for the training, development or operation of artificial intelligence (AI) technologies, including generative AI technologies. The rights holders expressly reserve this publication from the text and data mining exception as per Article 4(3) of the Digital Single Market Directive (EU) 2019/790.

Bloomsbury Publishing Inc does not have any control over, or responsibility for, any third-party websites referred to or in this book. All internet addresses given in this book were correct at the time of going to press. The author and publisher regret any inconvenience caused if addresses have changed or sites have ceased to exist, but can accept no responsibility for any such changes.

Library of Congress Cataloging-in-Publication Data
Names: Manns, Jessica (Embryologist) author
Title: The trying time : a comprehensive guide to infertility, IVF and family building / Jessica Manns.
Description: New York : Bloomsbury Academic, 2025. |
Includes bibliographical references and index.
Identifiers: LCCN 2025027680 (print) | LCCN 2025027681 (ebook) |
ISBN 9798881807351 hardback | ISBN 9798881807368 epub |
ISBN 9798881867553 adobe pdf
Subjects: LCSH: Infertility | Infertility—Treatment |
Fertilization in vitro, Human | Fertility clinics
Classification: LCC RC889 .M3644 2025 (print) | LCC RC889 (ebook)
LC record available at https://lccn.loc.gov/2025027680
LC ebook record available at https://lccn.loc.gov/2025027681

ISBN: HB: 979-8-8818-0735-1
ePDF: 979-8-8818-6755-3
eBook: 979-8-8818-0736-8

Typeset by Deanta Global Publishing Services, Chennai, India
Printed and bound in the United States of America

For product safety related questions contact productsafety@bloomsbury.com.

To find out more about our authors and books visit www.bloomsbury.com and sign up for our newsletters.

Contents

Acknowledgments vi
Preface vii

1 Infertility Trauma and Support 1

2 Male Reproduction and Infertility 13

3 Female Reproduction and Infertility 27

4 Meeting Your Fertility Specialist 45

5 Diagnostic Tests and Treatment Options 51

6 Fertility Medications and IVF Monitoring 65

7 In Vitro Fertilization (IVF) 77

8 Preimplantation Genetic Testing (PGT) 135

9 Failed Implantation and Pregnancy Loss 151

10 Coping with Loss and Grief 173

11 Optimizing Reproductive Health 191

12 Third-Party Reproduction 205

13 Nurturing Supportive Relationships 235

Directory of Contributors 241
Glossary of Terms and Abbreviations 248
Notes 254
Index 265

Acknowledgments

This guide would not have been made possible without the amazing contributors who voluntarily donated their professional or personal stories. Thank you to my manager, Liz Heijkoop, and literary agent, Joëlle Delbourgo. A special thank you to my cousin, River Wintermantel, for creating many of the graphics within the guide. And to my husband, who encouraged me to keep going from the moment I mentioned to him the idea of creating this guide.

Preface

If you or someone you know has experienced infertility, you likely understand that it is often a painstaking and uphill journey with financial, physical, mental, and emotional tolls. It can be deeply isolating and may have significant and lasting impacts on self-esteem and relationships.

With one in six people worldwide experiencing infertility in their lifetime, infertility directly and indirectly affects millions. These numbers are staggering and will continue to rise over time. And, while there is no universally-accepted definition of infertility, major health organizations often use limited definitions that exclude many individuals from receiving the diagnosis and care they need to build their families in a timely manner. For example, the World Health Organization (WHO) currently defines infertility as a disease of the male or female reproductive system, characterized by the failure to achieve a pregnancy after twelve months or more of regular, unprotected sexual intercourse. This antiquated and arbitrary definition excludes not only those who can conceive but are unable to carry a pregnancy to term, but also members of the LGBTQ+ community and single parents. In fact, some countries have policies that prohibit fertility treatment for same-sex couples, single parents, and unmarried couples. Other countries prohibit or restrict the use of donor sperm, donor eggs, donor embryos, or gestational carriers (surrogates). Policies change all the time, so it's important to stay informed about the current policies in the area in which you plan to undergo fertility treatment.

Moreover, this definition fails to consider that many people across the world are waiting longer to have children for personal, medical, or professional reasons. Fertility declines with age, so requiring a year of unprotected intercourse can waste precious time in which fertility treatment such as in vitro fertilization (IVF) can be completed. For this reason, some health organizations have altered their definitions of infertility, stating that a couple is considered infertile if they're unable to conceive after six months of regular, unprotected sexual intercourse when the female partner is 35 or older. Further, some individuals are unable to conceive via sexual intercourse due to medical reasons such as blocked fallopian tubes or azoospermia (no sperm in the ejaculate), regardless of how long they try to conceive. Can you imagine how people must feel when they learn that they have wasted months or years trying to conceive with a condition that makes conception through intercourse nearly impossible?

It's also worth noting that fertility treatment is very expensive. While some public funds and insurance policies cover some or all of the costs associated with these treatments, others do not cover any of the costs or only cover costs for those who meet specific eligibility requirements. When coverage is unavailable, it is often difficult or even impossible to pay for the associated costs, and many people must make difficult financial decisions in order to afford a chance (but not a guarantee) to build their families. Where coverage is lacking, great strides must be made to make fertility treatment affordable and accessible for all.

In 2023, a significant event occurred in the United States: the American Society for Reproductive Medicine (ASRM) altered its long-standing definition of infertility, which it now defines as[1]:

a disease, condition, or status characterized by any of the following:

- *The inability to achieve a successful pregnancy based on a patient's medical, sexual, and reproductive history, age, physical findings, diagnostic testing, or any combination of those factors.*
- *The need for medical intervention, including, but not limited to, the use of donor gametes or donor embryos in order to achieve a successful pregnancy either as an individual or with a partner.*
- *In patients having regular, unprotected intercourse and without any known etiology for either partner suggestive of impaired reproductive ability, evaluation should be initiated at 12 months when the female partner is under 35 years of age and at six months when the female partner is 35 years of age or older.*

Nothing in this definition shall be used to deny or delay treatment to any individual, regardless of relationship status or sexual orientation.

My hope is that a universal definition of infertility will emerge that is inclusive and ensures access to all family-building options, regardless of where someone lives. It will take time to break certain barriers and there will be resistance, but even small steps toward progress can lead to meaningful change.

A Need for Awareness and Education

For years, infertility was a taboo topic, and many people suffered in silence. Even today, some choose to keep their journeys private for a number of reasons. Further, there were limited resources available regarding IVF and infertility until recently. Many people were (and still are) left feeling isolated and in the dark wondering why they couldn't get pregnant when it seemed that everyone around them could do so without any issues.

Infertility awareness and advocacy remind people that they are not alone in their struggles, destigmatize infertility, encourage open conversations about infertility, help enforce changes in laws and policies that improve access to fertility treatments, normalize diverse paths to parenthood, and empower people to seek treatment in a timely manner. Fortunately, there have been advancements in infertility awareness and advocacy. More people, including celebrities, are sharing their struggles with infertility, making it less taboo and creating a space where people feel less isolated through their journeys. Many movies and television shows now include infertility storylines. A growing number of virtual and in-person infertility support groups are now available. More people are taking proactive steps to optimize and preserve their fertility at younger ages. And in some regions, policies are changing to make fertility treatment more accessible.

Education is equally important. It empowers people to make informed decisions about their reproductive health and treatment options, promotes effective healthcare practices, and challenges misconceptions about infertility, IVF, and various family-building options.

Today, there are many excellent educational resources available for anyone desiring more information about infertility, fertility treatments, and family-building options in the form of social media, websites, and apps. However, many of these resources are difficult to understand and often present conflicting information, which can cause mental and emotional exhaustion (I think we've all been guilty of falling down the "Google rabbit hole" at some point).

But everyone should be able to understand this important information. We need to recognize that, despite what we learned in high school, it's not always easy to get pregnant. Anyone trying to conceive or seeking fertility treatment should have a basic understanding of the reproductive systems, common causes of infertility and pregnancy loss, available treatment options, methods for optimizing fertility, and the mental and emotional tolls of infertility and fertility treatment. And those who desire or need to pursue third-party reproduction or adoption should have access to educational resources about these paths to parenthood. Knowledge is power, after all.

This is why there is a need for this all-inclusive, easily accessible guide to IVF (and other fertility treatments), infertility, and family-building options. When I began working on it, I knew the topics that I wanted the guide to cover, **but I knew that I couldn't write it alone.** I am not a doctor, nurse, mental health specialist, or genetic counselor, so I reached out to those who are. I was overwhelmed at how many amazing professionals agreed to *voluntarily* contribute valuable information about some very complex topics. This guide wouldn't exist without their help, and they deserve immense credit for its success. With their help, each chapter contains important, evidence-based information written in a manner that is easy to understand.

However, even with these outstanding professional contributions, the guide needed one more important element: a personal touch. So, I asked my Instagram followers to share their stories and explain how their experiences can help others. Again, the response was overwhelming. My hope is that you find a story or two in this guide that resonates with you, helps you through your journey, and reminds you that you are not alone.

The Guide's Layout

First, who is this guide written for? The short answer is: anyone. However, it will be especially helpful for those at any stage of their fertility journeys, as well as anyone who wants more information about IVF, infertility, and family-building options. This might include aspiring medical professionals, loved ones who want to offer support, and those who are interested in preserving their fertility or considering adoption.

The guide begins with a crucial topic: infertility and mental health. Many people don't realize the profound impact that infertility has on self-esteem and relationships. Learning to recognize these impacts and cope with the mental and emotional stress of infertility trauma can help individuals feel less isolated and more empowered to seek support.

We then dive into foundational knowledge about the male and female reproductive systems, including common causes of infertility. A basic understanding of how these sytems function is essential to grasp the underlying causes of infertility.

From there, we discuss some of the common first steps when seeking fertility treatment such as the first fertility consultation, a basic fertility workup, and other common diagnostic tests. The guide then provides detailed information about fertility treatment options, including IVF and preimplantation genetic testing (PGT). These chapters are packed with essential insights to guide you through each stage of the process.

We then shift the focus to possible causes of failed implantation and pregnancy loss. An entire chapter is also devoted to coping with loss, which, despite its importance, is sadly often reduced to a few sentences in most resources.

The following chapter focuses on methods for optimizing fertility outcomes that are supported by cited research studies. This is one of the hottest topics when it comes to infertility, and no details are spared about what to do (and what to avoid) to optimize your chances of success.

The focus then shifts to third-party reproduction and adoption. The sections in this chapter include information about donor sperm, donor eggs, donor embryos, surrogacy, and domestic infant adoption.

And the final chapter offers advice for supporting someone struggling with infertility. This chapter was added by request but is absolutely vital for this guide, and my hope is that it helps strengthen relationships between those who are struggling and their loved ones.

At the back of the book, you'll find a directory of all the professionals who contributed to the guide, a bibliography, a glossary of important terms, and an index.

Thank you for picking up this guide and taking the time to read through it. The culmination of professional and personal contributions truly makes this guide a unique and invaluable resource. I hope that you find it helpful and it encompasses all the information you need.

Sincerely,
Jessica

A note about wording in this guide:

Important notes

- Inclusive language and representation. I strive to use inclusive vocabulary throughout this guide in recognition and respect of all gender identities. However, due to the topics in this guide such as reproductive physiology, you may notice the following used interchangeably:

  - She/her/hers pronouns, woman/women, female, assigned female at birth (XX sex chromosomes and female reproductive organs at birth)
  - He/him/his pronouns, man/men, male, assigned male at birth (XY sex chromosomes and male reproductive organs at birth)

- Important medical disclaimer: I am not a licensed medical professional. The information provided in this guide is intended for general educational purposes only. It is not a substitute for professional medical advice, diagnosis, or treatment. Always consult your personal healthcare provider regarding any medical concerns or before making any health-related decisions.

- A note about mental health: infertility and loss can cause a wide range of emotions. If you or someone you know is exhibiting signs of clinical depression, anxiety, or trauma responses, please seek professional help. You do not have to suffer in silence.

Chapter 1
Infertility Trauma and Support

The information in this chapter was contributed by Chiemi Rajamahendran (Miss.Conception Coach), infertility trauma and loss support specialist

When we are young, we are taught how to avoid getting pregnant, but we're rarely taught that conceiving a child is sometimes a challenging or impossible process. For many, the inability to conceive is a heartbreaking and traumatic experience that affects multiple aspects of their lives. In fact, the term *infertility trauma* is now widely used to describe the emotional, mental, and physical tolls that infertility can take on one's self-esteem and relationships. Though nearly 17 percent of people worldwide will experience infertility in their lifetimes, it often remains a silent struggle.

This chapter explores the causes and signs of infertility trauma, as well as how it affects internal and external relationships. It's important to remember that everyone has a unique experience and reaction to infertility trauma, and all of these reactions are valid. Infertility trauma should be taken seriously, and there are a number of resources (described below) available for anyone in need of support.

There are many causes of infertility trauma, including:

- Compounding Emotions. Infertility trauma is often described as a form of complex trauma—not one singular event, but a series of emotionally overwhelming experiences that accumulate over time. Some individuals or couples wait months or even years before they receive an infertility diagnosis and/or begin fertility treatment. In the meantime, they are consistently left heartbroken as each menstrual cycle ends with a period instead of a pregnancy. Often, there's little time to pause or process these feelings. Instead, the focus shifts immediately to the next cycle, the next attempt, the next possibility. Over time, this cycle of hope and disappointment creates a buildup of unresolved grief, anxiety, and emotional fatigue that can affect their quality of life.

- Loss of Hope. Infertility can be a roller coaster of emotions ranging from hopefulness to hopelessness in a short period of time. *Thus, infertility itself is a loss.* It's the gradual loss of a dream and expectation that, over many months or years, can cause a profound loss of hope.
- Too Many Unknowns. Those experiencing infertility trauma are often left wondering why they cannot get pregnant as easily as others. They often must also alter their projected timelines, such as when they will build their families, for indefinite amounts of time without knowing if and when their dreams will come true. During this time, many questions frustratingly go unanswered, such as:
  - Why is this happening to me/us?
  - What are we doing wrong?
  - Where should we go from here?
- Sacrificing So Much. Sometimes, infertility trauma comes from feeling like you've already had to sacrifice so much (the fun planning, spur of the moment sex, anticipation of the two-week wait, excitement of a first pregnancy test) only to be left without a pregnancy.
- Feeling Powerless. Receiving an infertility diagnosis and undergoing fertility treatment can also be very traumatic because these experiences consist of procedures, tests, appointments, schedules, protocols, and dynamics with healthcare professionals. Each of these can leave one feeling powerless and vulnerable. The time commitment alone can disrupt careers, strain relationships, and interfere with personal milestones. Vacations are postponed, life events are rescheduled, and the sense of control over one's future begins to slip away.
- Financial Strain. Fertility treatment (especially IVF) can be very expensive and have lasting financial impacts, especially in areas where treatment isn't covered. In fact, many people who would benefit from fertility treatment do not pursue it due to the costs. Others take out loans, refinance their homes, or work multiple jobs to afford treatment. Sadly, fertility treatment does not guarantee a successful outcome, and many people must undergo multiple treatment cycles.

- Feeling Inadequate. Infertility can lead to feelings of inadequacy, guilt, and shame. These emotions often intensify when they see others getting pregnant effortlessly ("all of our friends are pregnant except for us."), which can intensify stress, diminish self-esteem, and strain relationships.
- Triggering Events. Pregnancy announcements, baby showers, and other milestones can evoke feelings of resentment, jealousy, anger, and sadness.
- Lack of Support. Infertility can be overwhelming, isolating, and depressing. Some people elect to not share their struggles with others, which can exacerbate these emotions. Others seek support through family members, friends, online communities, or professionals. However, even with a small or large support system, feelings of loneliness and emotional exhaustion may persist. In many cases, additional help from a licensed mental health professional may be required.
- Other Causes. Infertility trauma can stem from various other causes, including:
  - Physical changes such as weight gain or bruising from fertility medications
  - Altered relationships with others
  - Loss of intimacy in relationships
  - Pressure from family members ("when are you going to give me a grandchild?")
  - Pregnancy loss at any stage

Recognizing Infertility Trauma

The truth is that no one ever communicates with one single emotion. So, infertility trauma can present as a smile, tears, or anything in between. Those struggling with infertility trauma feel in circles, not straight lines, and their emotions learn to coexist. It's normal to laugh one minute and cry the next, to feel strong one moment and then second-guess everything they thought they'd learned the following.

Some common emotions during this time may include:

- Guilt ("it's my fault we can't get pregnant")
- Angry ("other people get pregnant without even trying")
- Shame ("others are counting on me to get pregnant, but I can't")

Symptoms from infertility trauma and related experiences are valid and real, though sometimes they don't even seem like symptoms. Common examples include:

- Irregular sleep patterns
- Insomnia
- Anxiety
- Worst-case scenario thinking
- Bouts of depression/isolation and anger from anxiety
- Weight gain or loss
- Fear of being touched or within close proximity of others
- Sensitivity to loud noises
- Feeling overwhelmed by big groups

Recognizing these feelings and symptoms can be difficult, but if you or someone you know is experiencing any of these while navigating infertility trauma, do not hesitate to seek support or professional help. You are not alone, and your experience is valid.

The Impact of Fertility Trauma on Self-Esteem

It is common for people to blame themselves when they are unable to conceive, especially when they receive an infertility diagnosis. Both men and women have reported that they feel inadequate or defective ("I can't even do the one thing that is supposed to be so natural."), and many experience shame, stress, anxiety, depression, and diminished self-esteem. Infertility can also lead to identity crises and strain external relationships ("why would anyone else want to be around me when I don't even want to be around myself?").

Though these feelings are common for both men and women, they are especially prevalent among women who are undergoing fertility treatment since the medications and procedures can cause side effects such as mood swings, temporary weight gain, and bruising that can continue even after treatment ends.

So, how do you cope with self-esteem issues?

While it's often easier said than done, it's important to remember these important truths:

- *Your infertility is not your fault.*
- *You are going through a difficult and temporary experience that will pass.*

- You are not alone in your struggles. More people experience infertility trauma than you might think.
- You don't need to hit rock bottom to be deserving of empathy.
- You are stronger than you think.
- You don't need to lose your sanity to accept emotional support.
- You don't need to be physically unwell to need time to rest and heal.
- These hard, complicated emotions are never a reflection of your character.
- Infertility doesn't have to be a lonely, isolating place.
- Hanging on by a thread doesn't have to be the norm.
- You are not meant to do this alone.
- Anger is a healthy part of the process.
- Infertility can make you question your faith.
- Infertility can feel all-consuming, and you may question your sanity.
- Hormones and medications can intensify your emotions.
- A positive pregnancy test doesn't erase all the anxiety.
- You have more control over this process than might realize.

If you're struggling with self-esteem issues related to infertility, try listening to your body's needs. It may help to ask yourself:

- What is my body feeling?
- What do I need?
- What do I want?
- What do I feel?

Try to practice self-care and treat yourself with kindness and understanding. When you are feeling overwhelmed, try using positive affirmations or journaling to express your thoughts. Activities such as outdoor walking or relaxation techniques like yoga can help clear your mind and manage stress. If you are feeling isolated or in need of additional support, it can help to reach out to loved ones, the online community, virtual or in-person support groups, or professionals who can help you express and process your emotions.

> ### Kendra's Story
>
> *I remember the first time the word infertility was used by my OB/GYN. My husband and I had been trying to conceive for six years on our own. Ovulation kits, laying around with my legs up in the air after intercourse, and feeling the pit in my stomach each month when my cycle started. When infertility was explained to me, I remember feeling that I lost my trust and faith that my husband and I would ever be parents.*
>
> *Throughout the six years of trying to conceive, the doctors identified small things that they believed could've been contributing to our inability to get pregnant. But once those areas were rectified and treated, month after month, we were still left with nothing.*
>
> *When given an infertility diagnosis, there's a change in how you see yourself and the world. Even though only a small percentage of people need to go the route of utilizing assisted reproductive technologies, it is stressful to think about whether or not that will be part of the plan. And sometimes there's a known cause, but sometimes there is not. Depending on what is contributing to the diagnosis, the layers of emotional distress can be very difficult to manage. Research has shown that people dealing with infertility have the same levels of stress and anxiety as someone dealing with cancer and heart disease. I think that says enough in itself to understand how difficult infertility can be. It is a loss. A loss of hopes, dreams, and self-identity. It's also a loss of what you thought your process to have a baby would look like. So, if you feel like you're going through this alone, you're not. It's more common than you think, and there are a lot of great resources available if you need them.*

The Impact of Fertility Trauma on Relationships with Partners

One of the most impactful effects of infertility trauma is its effect on the relationship between partners. The reality is that infertility is often a new (and huge) experience, and most couples do not know how to navigate it together. And, for many couples, infertility is the first challenge they will face individually and/or as a couple. Infertility trauma can bring out both the best and the most difficult aspects of a relationship.

If you are trying to conceive with your partner, your intimacy may be impacted. Many couples enter relationships expecting to build a family through an intimate experience, but infertility can alter that expectation. Over time, sex may begin to feel like a regimented, mandated task required by medical professionals. It can become difficult to separate sex for pleasure or intimacy versus sex for fertility treatment purposes. In the case of IVF, sex is not even required in order to conceive a pregnancy. Unfortunately, this can affect couples even after a pregnancy occurs.

Beyond intimacy, infertility trauma can mentally and emotionally affect your relationship with your partner because you are both carrying a heavy emotional load. This is especially true if you are not sharing your experience with others Here are some common ways this strain can manifest:

- You are experiencing heavy emotions but do not want to burden your partner, so you keep your emotions bottled up. Your partner does not realize how overwhelmed you feel and does not know how to support you. Eventually, you may feel abandoned and resent your partner for his/her lack of comfort and support.

- You and your partner are constantly feeling stressed and emotionally drained. You try not to focus on your infertility, but it's always in the back of your mind. It becomes increasingly difficult to enjoy spending time together because you are both on edge all of the time.

- Women undergoing fertility treatment often cannot physically detach themselves from treatment and recovery, so they may feel that the weight is all being carried on their shoulders. But this is not true; partners are also navigating their own emotional experience. In some situations, a partner may innately feel helpless or guilty for not being able to share the physical load.

- It may be difficult for you to open up about your struggles because it makes you feel vulnerable. Instead, you shut down and become isolated from your partner.

<u>Is it possible to maintain a healthy relationship throughout this time?</u>

Absolutely. In fact, many couples find that infertility strengthens their relationship. It's very important that you and your partner maintain open, honest communication and mutual support throughout your journey, keeping in mind that some days may be more difficult than others. Here are some ways to nurture your relationship and combat the effects of infertility trauma:

- Talk with your partner about your definitions of intimacy. Your definition may need to shift a little while you are trying to conceive, but intimacy itself does not need to disappear. For example, you can think of intimacy as cuddling on the couch while watching a movie or going out on a date together. You can also consider only one room in your house a "baby-making room" and keep other spaces reserved for connection and comfort. Remember that there are both physical and psychological aspects of intimacy, and try not to lose sight of your commitment and love for one another in the process.

- Tell your partner exactly what you need so he/she knows how to support you, and ask how you can support him/her. Remember that everyone deals with stress differently and your needs can change in a matter of days or even hours.
- Remind yourself and your partner why you fell in love. You are more than a couple trying to get pregnant. You are partners in life.
- Normalize and acknowledge that you are going through or have been through a challenging experience, and this experience will not last forever. Infertility is a journey, not a destination.
- Take a walk and talk to your partner about what is making you angry, fearful, or resentful. This can help remind you that you're working toward the same goal together.
- Discuss your options with your partner. Do you both want to continue trying to conceive every month? Do you feel the need to take a break from trying? Are you ready to consult a fertility specialist?
- If you are struggling to communicate about complex emotions, try to break down your emotions with your partner one piece at a time. For example, share how something that your partner did made you feel. This may feel uncomfortable at first, especially if you are not used to relaying what you want and choosing your own needs. Keep in mind that some of your feelings may not make sense, and that's okay. This process can take time.
- Seek professional support if needed. A counselor or therapist can help you and your partner navigate the emotional terrain of infertility and strengthen your communication.

The Impact of Fertility Trauma on Relationships with Others

Aside from your partner, infertility trauma can have a huge effect on your relationships with others, including your family members, friends, and coworkers. If you choose to share your journey with others, you may not receive the support or validation that you need. This can create awkward dynamics, which may cause you to form emotional boundaries to protect yourself. This is especially true if you feel any family pressure to have children ("when are you going to give me a grandchild?") or if you are trying to respect family dynamics to make others happy (like attending a baby shower for a family member). It's okay to decline invitations to events that might be triggering. It may also help to have an exit plan in place if you want to leave an uncomfortable social situation. Do not force yourself to remain in any situation that makes you feel frustrated or upset.

In some situations, others may unintentionally make hurtful comments or offer unsolicited advice, which can intensify your emotions. If you are comfortable doing so, calmly explain why their remarks are hurtful or unnecessary to help prevent similar situations in the future. If you are uncomfortable speaking up, calmly leave the conversation (or the event altogether) and allow yourself to process any feelings associated with their remarks when you are in a safe space. Talking with a support person or professional about these encounters can also be helpful.

Infertility trauma can be especially difficult if your friends are having children and engaging in family activities and traditions. This can cause feelings of jealousy and resentment even if you are genuinely happy for them. If this happens, try asking your friends for an adults-only night out. Alternatively, consider reaching out to others within the infertility community who understand what you are experiencing and are going through similar struggles. This can lead to new friendships and an added layer of support throughout your journey.

Infertility Trauma Resources

Though it might seem difficult at first, one of the easiest ways to heal from infertility trauma is to connect with others. This could mean following social media accounts (you can make an anonymous account to keep your journey private), attending virtual or in-person support groups, or talking to a professional such as an infertility counselor.

Renee's Story

We started trying to have a baby when I was thirty-one. At age thirty-three, I was unexpectedly diagnosed with severe diminished ovarian reserve and suspected endometriosis. No one in my family had struggled to conceive and I did not personally know anyone who had been through infertility, so I felt completely blindsided when it happened to me. We ended up doing an IVF

> cycle, which ended in a miscarriage, and were left with little hope. Infertility and pregnancy loss were the hardest things I had ever been through and IVF felt so overwhelming.
>
> I didn't know where to turn or who to talk to, and it just felt like people were often saying all of the wrong things to me. I created an anonymous account on Instagram and started documenting our journey and connecting with others online who were also going through similar journeys. Suddenly, I felt so much less isolated. I learned so much and always had someone to talk to who really "got it." I wish I had found that beautiful online community even earlier! My mental health greatly improved after finding this support system.

Support is about learning tools and techniques that allow for subtle, meaningful shifts. It provides you with a safe place to share, be seen, and feel validated in a non-judgmental environment. It also helps you establish a sense of control, which is essential to feel safe.

When it comes to infertility counseling, the goal is to help you feel understood and equipped with tools to help process emotions as they arise. Ultimately, infertility counselors support those trying to conceive by exploring the roots of emotions like jealousy, anger and disconnection, and work through how these feelings show up in daily life. They understand that trying to conceive can be frustrating, scary, and extremely lonely at times. An infertility counselor aims to help you:

- manage your painful feelings;
- normalize your behavior (because *all behavior makes sense in the context of infertility trauma*);
- shift the weight of your experiences;
- recognize and process what are genuine emotions versus what are trauma reactions. These feelings are all-consuming, overwhelming, and can sometimes cloud your judgment or challenge your beliefs;
- work through tough emotions and hard decisions;
- feel better in your day-to-day life;
- gain more control over your life;
- work through the trauma you've experienced and may still be carrying;
- gain new perspectives and tools to live with more peace moving forward.

Conclusions

Infertility can have profound emotional, mental, and physical impacts on your self-esteem and relationships with others. It is important to establish a support system to prevent isolation and process your thoughts and emotions, whether it is through a support person, online community, support group, or professional. Infertility trauma is very real, and all associated emotions are valid.

Chapter 2
Male Reproduction and Infertility

The information in this chapter was contributed by Justin Houman, MD, men's health urologist and fellowship-trained male reproductive medicine and surgery specialist.

The male reproductive system is responsible for producing and delivering sperm for fertilization of the female egg. Understanding the anatomy and physiology of the male reproductive system can help you better understand how reproduction works and how certain abnormalities can contribute to male factor infertility (MFI).

Anatomy of the Male Reproductive System

The male reproductive system is made up of several organs and structures (Figure 2.1), including the:

- **Testes (testicle):** two small, oval-shaped organs located in the scrotum (a muscular sac surrounded by a layer of skin) outside of the body. They are responsible for producing sperm and the hormone testosterone. The testes consist of small, coiled seminiferous tubules.
- **Epididymis:** a long, coiled tube that connects to the testes and stores and matures the sperm.

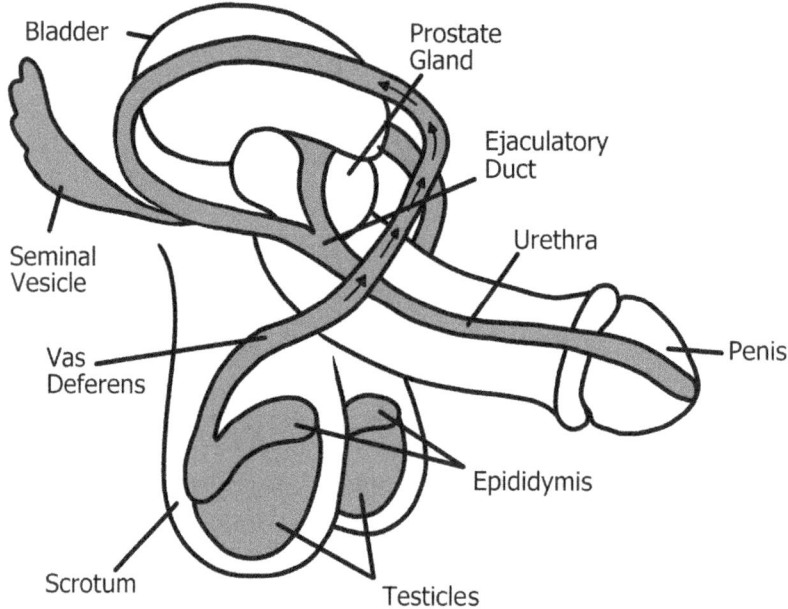

Figure 2.1 The anatomy of the male reproductive system.

- **Vas Deferens:** a muscular tube that carries sperm from the epididymis to the urethra.
- **Seminal vesicles and prostate gland:** glands that produce fluids that mix with the sperm to form semen.
- **Ejaculatory ducts:** paired tubes that form where the vas deferens meets the seminal vesicles. They travel through the prostate gland and connect to the urethra.
- **Urethra:** the tube inside of the penis that carries semen and urine out of the body.

Physiology of Male Reproduction

The male reproductive system is regulated by hormones produced in the brain and the testes. These hormones control the production and release of sperm and testosterone in the testes.

Spermatogenesis (sperm production) begins at puberty when the anterior pituitary gland in the brain releases follicle-stimulating hormone (FSH) and luteinizing hormone (LH). These hormones travel to the testes, where FSH stimulates sperm production and LH stimulates testosterone production. Testosterone is required for sperm production but also plays a crucial role in the development and maintenance of male physical characteristics, such as facial hair.

Sperm production occurs within Sertoli cells, located in the coiled seminiferous tubules of the testes. Sperm production is temperature-sensitive, which is why it occurs in the testes (which are slightly cooler than core body temperature). Within these cells, sperm divide and differentiate into immature, non-motile sperm cells. Once formed, they travel to the epididymis, where they mature and gain the ability to swim and fertilize an egg. Mature sperm are stored in the epididymis until ejaculation.

During sexual arousal, the muscles in the vas deferens and prostate gland contract, propelling the sperm through the reproductive tract. During this time, sperm are bathed in fluids from the prostate gland and seminal vesicles, forming a substance known as semen. This mixture is then expelled through the urethra and out of the body during ejaculation.

Anatomy and Physiology of Sperm

Spermatozoa (sperm) are the male gametes, or sex cells, that fertilize oocytes (eggs) during conception. They consist of a(n):

- **Acrosome**: cap-like structure on the sperm's head that contains the enzyme hyaluronidase, which is essential for penetrating the cells and shell surrounding an egg
- **Head**: contains the sperm's genetic material (DNA) within its nucleus
- **Midpiece**: packed with mitochondria, which provide energy for the sperm to move and fertilize an egg
- **Tail (flagellum):** enables the sperm to move toward the egg

When sperm enter the female reproductive tract, they travel to the egg inside of the fallopian tube. During this time, they undergo a series of changes known as capacitation, which prepare them to fertilize the egg (during fertility treatment, capacitation occurs outside of the body prior to insemination). As sperm approach the egg, they release the enzymes from their acrosomes to break through the cells surrounding the egg and penetrate the egg's shell. One sperm

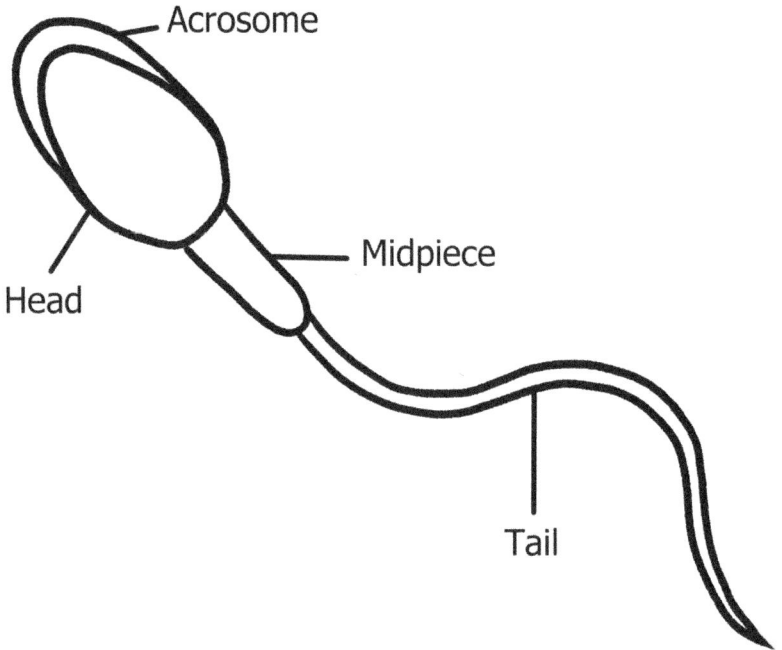

Figure 2.2 The anatomy of a spermatozoa (sperm).

ultimately penetrates the shell and fuses with the egg's inner plasma membrane, triggering a reaction (block to polyspermy) that prevents additional sperm from entering the egg. The sperm then deposits its DNA into the egg, initiating a series of events to occur that can result in fertilization of the egg. See Chapter 3 for more information about this process.

Male Factor Infertility

Male factor infertility (MFI) refers to conditions that affect a male's ability to conceive a pregnancy. These issues can arise from various factors that affect sperm production, transport, or function. It is estimated that male infertility accounts for roughly 33 percent of infertility cases. Understanding the common conditions associated with MFI is crucial in diagnosing and effectively managing infertility issues in men. Timely diagnosis, appropriate treatment, and assisted reproductive techniques can help overcome these challenges and improve fertility outcomes. By exploring the causes, impact, and treatment options for MFI, individuals and healthcare providers can work together to address MFI and support those on their journeys to parenthood.

There are several disorders and abnormalities that can contribute to MFI, including:

1. Varicocele is a condition in which the veins in the scrotum become enlarged and twisted, which can affect sperm production by:

- Decreasing blood flow to the testes
- Increasing the temperature in the testes
- Increasing the presence of reactive oxidative species (ROS), which can cause oxidative stress and sperm DNA damage

Varicocele is the most common correctable cause of MFI, affecting approximately 1 in 6 men of reproductive age in the general population. Forty percent of men diagnosed with infertility have varicoceles. It can be diagnosed through a physical or, less commonly, ultrasound examination.

If varicocele is affecting one's fertility, treatment options typically involve:

- **Varicocelectomy**: surgery to remove or repair the affected veins
- **Embolization**: a small coil or balloon is inserted into the affected vein to block blood flow, which forces blood to travel through the unaffected veins

Studies have shown that surgical treatment of varicocele can improve sperm count, motility, and morphology, and may increase the chances of natural conception or success with IUI or IVF.[1] It may also reduce sperm DNA fragmentation, though more research is needed.

2. Azoospermia is a condition in which there is no sperm in the semen. This can be caused by a blockage in the reproductive tract (obstructive azoospermia) or a problem with sperm production (non-obstructive azoospermia).

Azoospermia affects approximately 1 percent of men in the general population. It is diagnosed if no sperm is present during two or more semen analyses.

Treatment for azoospermia depends on the underlying cause. If there is a blockage, surgery may be required to remove the blockage, or sperm can be obtained through a procedure that collects sperm before they encounter the blockage. For example, sperm retrieval techniques such as testicular sperm extraction (TESE) or microdissection testicular sperm extraction (micro-TESE) may be an option to retrieve viable sperm from the testes for use in IVF. For non-obstructive azoospermia, hormone therapy may be required to promote sperm production. In most of these cases, IVF with ICSI (intracytoplasmic sperm injection) is required for fertilization. In some situations, it unfortunately may not be possible to treat non-obstructive azoospermia even with hormone therapy.

3. Oligospermia is a condition in which there are abnormally low levels of sperm in the semen. This can be caused by a variety of factors, including hormonal imbalances, varicocele, genetic disorders such as Klinefelter syndrome, infections, and environmental factors such as exposure to toxins or radiation. Oligospermia affects fertility because less sperm are ejaculated and are able to reach the egg to achieve fertilization.

Oligospermia affects approximately 30 percent of infertile men. It is often diagnosed via a semen analysis, though hormone and genetic tests may also be performed if needed.

Treatment for oligospermia depends on the underlying cause. In some cases, lifestyle changes such as quitting smoking, reducing alcohol intake, and improving diet and exercise habits can help improve sperm count and motility. Additionally, antibiotics (if an infection is present) or medications that stimulate sperm production, such as clomiphene citrate or gonadotropins, may be used to treat oligospermia. In cases where medication and lifestyle changes are not effective, IVF with ICSI may be used to improve the chances of successful fertilization for those with oligospermia. Certain genetic disorders cannot be treated.

4. **Teratospermia (Teratozoospermia)** refers to abnormal sperm morphology, where a significant portion of the sperm exhibit structural defects in the head, midpiece, or tail. These abnormalities can hinder the ability of sperm to fertilize an egg because it affects motility and the sperm's ability to penetrate the egg's protective layers, which reduces the chances of successful conception.

Teratospermia can be caused by genetic factors, environmental exposures to toxins or radiation, infections, hormonal imbalances, lifestyle habits such as smoking or excessive alcohol consumption, chronic stress, or overheating of the testes (e.g., from laptops). Varicocele is also associated with teratospermia.

Teratospermia is diagnosed via a semen analysis. In these cases, less than 4 percent of the sperm in a semen sample have normal morphology.

Treatment options for teratospermia depend on the severity of the condition. Mild cases may still allow for natural conception, while more severe cases might require assisted reproductive techniques such as IVF with ICSI. Lifestyle changes such as maintaining a healthy diet and exercise plan, avoiding smoking and excessive alcohol consumption, and minimizing exposure to toxins and prolonged heat may help improve sperm morphology.

5. **Oligoasthenoteratospermia (OAT)** refers to a combination of a low sperm count, decreased or absent motility, and abnormal morphology. It can result from genetic factors, DNA damage in sperm cells, hormonal imbalances, varicocele, chronic infections, testicular injury or inflammation, exposure to toxins or radiation, smoking, excessive alcohol consumption, drug use, poor diet, obesity, certain medications, or prolonged heat exposure to the testicles.

OAT is diagnosed through a semen sample. Natural conception with OAT can be very difficult, especially in severe cases. Treatment depends on the underlying cause but might include lifestyle modifications or hormone therapy. IVF with ICSI is typically recommended to increase the chances of fertilization.

6. **Retrograde ejaculation** occurs when semen flows backward into the bladder instead of being expelled through the penis during ejaculation. Usually, the opening to the bladder is closed off during an ejaculation to prevent sperm from entering it, which forces the sperm out of the body. However, impaired bladder neck function or damage to the nerves that control ejaculation can cause semen to enter the bladder. Various factors can lead to retrograde ejaculation, including diabetes, surgery involving the bladder or prostate, certain medications, and neurological disorders such as multiple sclerosis.

Retrograde ejaculation can significantly affect fertility outcomes as sperm is not ejaculated into the female reproductive tract, reducing the chances of successful conception. However, sperm can still be retrieved from the urine and used for fertility treatments.

Retrograde ejaculation may be suspected if two ejaculations produce little to no semen. A diagnosis is confirmed if semen is present in a urine sample.

Treatment options for retrograde ejaculation depend on the underlying cause. Medications such as alpha-adrenergic agonists can help close the bladder neck and prevent semen from entering the bladder. If medications are ineffective, sperm retrieval techniques combined with assisted reproduction such as IVF with ICSI can be used.

7. **Hypogonadism** is a condition in which the testes produce insufficient or no testosterone, the primary male sex hormone. It can be classified as primary (the testicles aren't producing testosterone) or secondary (the brain isn't producing the hormones required for testosterone production). It impacts 40 percent of men over the age of forty-five and increases in prevalence with age. Hypogonadism often leads to impaired testosterone and sperm production, reducing fertility potential. Low testosterone levels can negatively impact sperm quantity, motility, and overall quality.

Primary hypogonadism can be caused by genetic conditions such as Klinefelter syndrome, undescended testes, testicular injury, chemotherapy or radiation, or certain infections. Secondary hypogonadism can result from hypothalamic or pituitary disorders, obesity, stress, or excessive exercise.

Hypogonadism is diagnosed via a blood test that measures the levels of pituitary and sex hormones in the blood.

Treatment options for hypogonadism involve testosterone replacement therapy (TRT) to restore testosterone levels. However, TRT may further suppress natural sperm production. In cases where fertility preservation is desired, alternative options such as gonadotropin therapy or selective estrogen receptor modulators (SERMs) can be used to stimulate sperm production while maintaining testosterone levels. In some cases, addressing lifestyle factors such as obesity can improve hypogonadism. When a pituitary tumor is present, shrinking or removing the tumor can treat hypogonadism.

8. **Cryptorchidism** is a condition characterized by undescended testes, where one or both testes fail to move from the abdomen into the scrotum during fetal development. In many cases, the teste(s) will descend without medical intervention within the first few months of life.

The exact causes of cryptorchidism are not fully understood, but it may involve genetic factors, hormonal imbalances, or prenatal factors such as maternal smoking or exposure to certain medications. About 3 percent of full-term male infants are born with cryptorchidism, while 30 percent of premature male infants are affected. Low birth weight is the primary risk factor.

Cryptorchidism can lead to impaired spermatogenesis due to the elevated temperature inside the abdomen, which is not conducive to normal sperm development. The higher temperatures can also reduce sperm motility, increase DNA damage, and induce apoptosis (programmed cell death). It also increases the risk of infertility and testicular cancer if not treated early.

Cryptorchidism is usually diagnosed through a physical examination. In these situations, testes cannot be located in one or either of the scrotal sacs. In some cases, an ultrasound examination may be required to determine the location of the undescended testes.

The standard treatment for cryptorchidism involves surgery called orchiopexy, which relocates the undescended testis into the scrotum. Early intervention, preferably before two years of age, is crucial for optimizing fertility outcomes.

9. **Erectile dysfunction (ED)**, also called impotence, refers to the consistent inability to achieve or maintain an erection sufficient for sexual intercourse. It affects around 40 percent of men at the age of forty, and increases in prevalence with age.

Physical causes include vascular diseases (e.g., atherosclerosis) that block blood flow to the penis, hormonal imbalances, neurological disorders, certain medications, and lifestyle factors like smoking, excessive alcohol consumption, lack of physical activity, or obesity. In addition, medical conditions such as diabetes and psychological factors such as anxiety, chronic stress, depression, or relationship problems can contribute to ED.

Erectile dysfunction can affect fertility outcomes by hindering vaginal penetration and ejaculation during sexual intercourse. However, it does not necessarily mean that viable sperm aren't being produced.

ED can be diagnosed through a comprehensive medical history evaluation, physical exam of the penis and testicles, blood test, or ultrasound. If physical causes are ruled out, a psychological evaluation may be performed to examine possible mental health conditions that are causing ED.

Treatment options for erectile dysfunction include lifestyle modifications, counseling, medications (e.g., phosphodiesterase-5 inhibitors), vacuum erection devices, penile implants, or, in some cases, surgery. Fertility treatments like IUI or IVF can also be used to achieve a pregnancy when natural conception is difficult or impossible due to ED.

10. **Andropause**, also known as late-onset hypogonadism, refers to the age-related decline in testosterone levels in men. It shares some similarities with menopause in women but occurs more gradually.

Andropause is primarily caused by age-related changes in the testes, resulting in decreased testosterone production. Other factors, such as obesity, chronic illness, and medications, can also contribute to declining testosterone levels. Additionally, there are some psychological causes of andropause, including depression and chronic stress.

While andropause is associated with reduced testosterone levels and a decline in overall fertility potential, men can still maintain some level of fertility until advanced age. However, sperm quantity and quality may decline, making conception more challenging.

Andropause is diagnosed via a blood test that measures testosterone and other reproductive hormone levels in the blood. In some cases, a physical or psychological evaluation may also be recommended to confirm the diagnosis.

Treatment options for andropause involve testosterone replacement therapy (TRT) to alleviate symptoms associated with low testosterone levels. However, TRT may negatively impact fertility by suppressing natural sperm production. Fertility preservation techniques, such as sperm cryopreservation, can be considered before starting TRT if fertility desires are present.

11. **Various genetic conditions** can cause abnormal sperm production, impaired sperm function, blocked transport of sperm, and abnormal development of the reproductive organs. Some may also increase the risk of testicular cancer.

Genetic conditions causing male infertility can be inherited or result from spontaneous genetic mutations. Examples include Klinefelter syndrome, Y chromosome microdeletions, cystic fibrosis gene mutations, and congenital absence of the vas deferens (CAVD).

Treatment options for genetic conditions causing male infertility depend on the specific condition and its underlying mechanisms. Assisted reproductive techniques such as IVF with ICSI combined with genetic testing of embryos (preimplantation genetic testing) may be used to select embryos free from the genetic condition. Genetic counseling is essential to provide information, guidance, and support to individuals and couples facing genetic causes of male infertility.

A Normal Semen Sample

Semen consists of sperm and fluid from the male reproductive tract. A normal semen sample typically contains millions of healthy, motile, and normally shaped sperm cells, though sperm make up only about 5 percent of a semen sample. The appearance and characteristics of a normal semen sample can vary depending on various factors such as age, lifestyle habits, and underlying health conditions. Understanding what constitutes a normal semen sample can help individuals and couples assess their fertility potential and identify any potential issues that may be affecting their ability to conceive. Note that some clinics will require multiple semen samples to diagnose MFI and may use different reference ranges (normal levels).

1. The total sperm count is the number of sperm present in a semen sample. In a normal sample, over 39 million sperm should be present, and at least 58 percent of the sperm should be alive. The sperm concentration refers to the number of sperm per milliliter (mL) of semen. Healthy males typically have at least 15 million sperm per milliliter of semen. A sperm concentration below this is considered low, which may indicate a reduced fertility potential since less sperm are able to reach and fertilize the egg.

2. Sperm motility refers to the ability of the sperm to move and swim through the female reproductive tract. A normal sperm sample should have at least 40 percent motile sperm, with 32 percent of the sperm having progressive motility, meaning they are able to swim forward in a relatively straight line. Poor sperm motility may result in difficulty reaching and fertilizing the egg.

3. Sperm morphology refers to the shape, size, and appearance of the sperm. A normal sperm sample should have at least 4 percent of sperm with normal morphology. Abnormal sperm morphology can be an indication of underlying health issues or genetic abnormalities that may affect fertility. Examples of abnormal sperm include those with large, small, or abnormally shaped heads, as well as those with two tails.

4. Other factors. In addition to sperm count, motility, and morphology, other factors can also be important in determining the health of a semen sample. For example, a normal semen volume is typically between 1.5 and 5 milliliters with a slightly alkaline pH level (7.2–8.0) that helps protect the sperm as they travel through the acidic female reproductive tract. The semen should liquify within 20-30 minutes and should have low or moderate viscosity. The presence of many white blood cells (>1 million per milliliter) in the sample may indicate infection or inflammation in the reproductive tract. There should be little to no agglutination (clumping of the sperm).

5. Advanced semen analysis results.

Sperm DNA fragmentation (SDF) refers to breaks or damage in a sperm's DNA. It has been associated with decreased rates of fertilization and embryo development. Further, embryos created from fragmented sperm are more likely to have damaged DNA, which can increase the chances of failed implantation and miscarriage.

SDF typically arises from oxidative stress due to infection, inflammation, varicocele, smoking, obesity, poor diet, excessive alcohol consumption, exposure to toxins or radiation, chemotherapy, and age. It can often be treated by reducing the factors that damage the DNA.

A sperm DNA fragmentation index (DFI) can determine the percentage of sperm within a semen sample with fragmented DNA. Typically, a semen sample with >30% fragmented sperm is considered abnormal, though ranges may vary between clinics. Unfortunately, there is no way to visualize DNA fragmentation prior to insemination, even with the use of ICSI. Men with very high sperm DFIs may opt for donor sperm to optimize their chances of success.

Antisperm antibodies (ASAs) are proteins produced by the male or female immune system that mistakenly attack and destroy sperm, which can reduce sperm count, motility, and transport through the female reproductive tract; capacitation and the acrosome reaction (processes necessary for fertilization); and sperm-egg interaction. ASAs may also impair fertilization, implantation, and embryo growth and development. They can be found in semen, blood, and female genital tract fluids such as cervical mucus.

In males, ASA production can be triggered by an infection or inflammation in the genital tract, sexually transmitted infections such as Chlamydia, or testicular injury or surgery. Chronic obstruction, such as a vasectomy reversal, can also lead to high and permanent ASA levels. In females, the exact cause of ASA production is less clear, but it may be related to an allergic reaction to semen.

For males, ASAs are often suspected when a semen analysis reveals a low sperm motility and/or high level of agglutination (clumping of sperm). ASAs can be diagnosed through tests including the Mixed Antiglobulin Reaction (MAR) blood test and the Immunobead Test (IBT) in a semen sample. For females, ASAs are most commonly detected via a blood sample, though cervical mucus or other fluid samples may also be required.

Treatment options for ASAs may include medication to lower the body's immune response, or fertility treatments such as intrauterine insemination (IUI) or IVF. Remember that, while ASA can impair conception, it's rare for antibodies alone to make pregnancy impossible.

Conclusions

Sperm production and release are regulated by hormones produced by the brain and testes. There are several disorders and abnormalities that can contribute to MFI. Treatment options vary depending on the underlying cause and severity of the condition, but may include surgery, hormone therapy, lifestyle changes, and fertility treatment. With proper treatment, successful reproductive outcomes are possible for many cases of MFI. A normal sperm sample typically contains millions of healthy, motile, and normally-shaped sperm cells. However, the appearance and characteristics of a normal semen sample can vary based on age, lifestyle habits, and overall health. If you are concerned about your fertility potential or experiencing difficulty conceiving, it is important to consult a healthcare provider to discuss potential causes and treatment options.

Shaun's Story

In 2017, my wife and I decided to start trying to expand our family and have children. We were so blissfully naive and assumed that we'd soon fall pregnant. But we didn't. After going to the GP (general practitioner) with our concerns and being referred for tests, it was established that I had no sperm (azoospermia).

Cue years of heartache, trauma, grief, failed operations, tough decisions, and even harder conversations, all of which was exacerbated for me by being a man. This time was spent feeling alone and dealing with a huge knock to my identity and ego.

But we got through it and, in 2021, we were blessed with twins born via the use of donor sperm. Life is good and full of love and laughter. I wouldn't change a thing about what I went through because it brought me to them.

When facing my darkest days of guilt and shame when faced with infertility, it was compounded by the fact that I couldn't find any other men talking about it. No one. So I thought I must be THE only one.

> *But I now know the statistics: that over 60 million men worldwide will face infertility, but there's still very few men talking about it. So I started sharing my story and putting my vulnerability out there on my Instagram account "Knackered Knackers" to let other men know that it's not just them, and that they can get through it.*

Chapter 3
Female Reproduction and Infertility

The information in this chapter was contributed by Catherine Gordon, MD, reproductive endocrinologist and infertility specialist.

Female Reproductive Anatomy

The female reproductive system is a complex network of organs that work together to support fertility and reproduction. Understanding the anatomy of this system is crucial for comprehending the biological processes that lead to conception and pregnancy. The primary organs involved in the female reproductive system are the ovaries, fallopian tubes, uterus, cervix, and vagina (Figure 3.1).

1. **Ovaries:** paired, almond-shaped organs located on either side of the uterus in the pelvis. Within the ovaries are thousands of follicles, fluid-filled structures that each house an immature egg (oocyte), which are created prior to birth.

The ovaries serve as the primary source of female reproductive hormones, including estradiol (E2, a form of estrogen) and progesterone (P4). E2 plays a key role in the development and maintenance of secondary sexual characteristics (e.g., breast development), regulation of the menstrual cycle, and preparation of the uterine lining for potential embryo implantation. After ovulation, the ovaries produce P4, which helps maintain the uterine lining and supports early pregnancy.

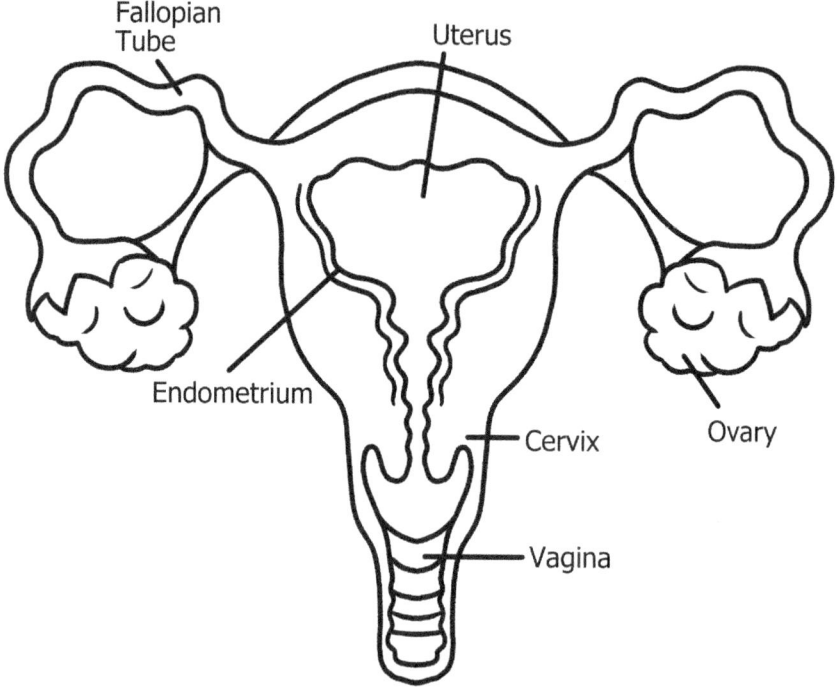

Figure 3.1 The anatomy of the female reproductive system.

2. **Fallopian tubes (oviducts):** bilateral tubes that extend from the area near the ovaries to the upper corners of the uterus. They play a vital role in capturing the ovulated egg, facilitating fertilization, and transporting the fertilized egg toward the uterus.

The tubes are approximately 10–14 centimeters long and divided into several segments:

- Infundibulum: the funnel-shaped, wider end of the fallopian tube closest to the ovary. It is surrounded by fingerlike projections called fimbriae, which sweep over the ovary during ovulation. The fimbriae capture the released egg from the ovary and guide it into the fallopian tube.
- Ampulla: the middle portion of the fallopian tube and is the site where fertilization most commonly occurs.

- Isthmus: the narrowest part of the fallopian tube, adjacent to the uterus. It connects the ampulla to the uterine cavity and facilitates the transport of sperm to the egg and the developing embryo to the uterus.

3. **Uterus:** a pear-shaped muscular organ where an embryo implants and develops into a fetus during pregnancy. It consists of three layers:

- Endometrium: The innermost layer that undergoes cyclic changes during the menstrual cycle in response to hormonal signals. If embryo implantation does not occur, the endometrial lining is shed during menstruation. If implantation does occur, the endometrium supports the implantation and development of the embryo.
- Myometrium: the middle layer composed of smooth muscle tissue. This muscular layer contracts during menstruation to expel menstrual fluid and during labor to facilitate childbirth.
- Perimetrium: the thin, outermost, protective layer that covers the surface of the uterus and connects it to surrounding structures.

4. **Cervix:** the lower, cylindrical portion of the uterus that forms a bridge between the uterine cavity and vaginal canal. It is composed of fibrous tissue, smooth muscle, and connective tissue, which provide structural support to the uterus and help regulate dilation and effacement during labor and childbirth. The cervix also acts as a physical barrier, protecting the upper reproductive tract from external contaminants and pathogens. It undergoes changes in response to hormonal fluctuations, allowing the passage of sperm during fertile periods while restricting access during non-fertile times.

4. **Vagina:** a flexible, muscular tube connecting the external genitalia (vulva) to the cervix. It is situated between the bladder and rectum, forming the lower portion of the birth canal. The external vaginal opening, or introitus, is located between the labia minora.

The vaginal canal varies in length among individuals but is typically around 6–7 inches long. Its muscular walls can expand and contract to accommodate sexual intercourse and childbirth. The vaginal environment is home to a delicate balance of microorganisms referred to as the vaginal flora. This balance is crucial for maintaining a healthy vaginal pH, which helps prevent infections, aids sperm motility on the journey to the cervix, and supports overall vaginal health.

The Menstrual Cycle

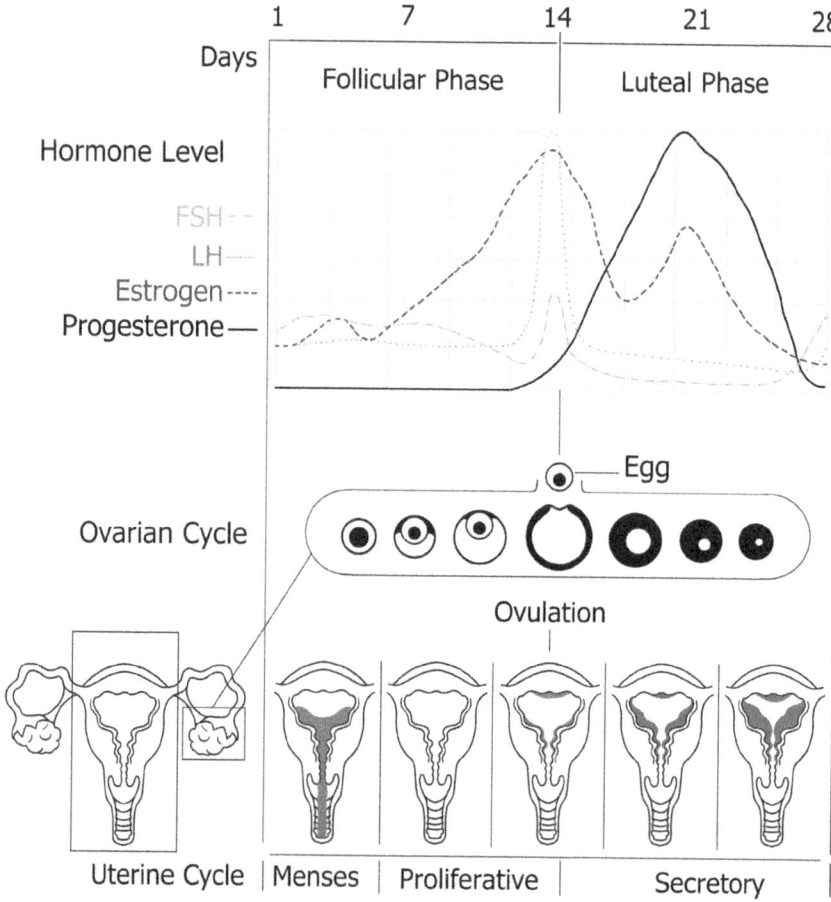

The menstrual cycle is a series of hormonal and physiological events that occur in the female body roughly every 28 days after puberty, though variations are common. It prepares the reproductive system for potential conception and pregnancy. The menstrual cycle consists of several phases: the menstrual phase, follicular phase, ovulation, and luteal phase.

1. **Menstrual phase:** This phase marks the beginning of the menstrual cycle and involves the shedding of the uterine lining (endometrium) if pregnancy did not occur during the previous cycle. Menstrual bleeding typically lasts around 3–7 days, though individual variations exist.

The menstrual phase is marked by low levels of estradiol (E2) and progesterone (P4), which were responsible for maintaining the uterine lining during the previous cycle. The decline in these hormones triggers the shedding of the uterine lining.

The shedding is a result of blood vessels constricting and then dilating, causing blood and tissue to be expelled from the uterus through the cervix and vagina.

Many individuals experience physical and emotional symptoms during the menstrual phase. Common symptoms include abdominal cramps (dysmenorrhea), bloating, breast tenderness, mood changes, and fatigue. These symptoms are often related to hormonal fluctuations and changes in the uterine lining.

2. **Follicular phase:** The follicular phase sets the stage for ovulation and potential conception. It typically lasts 10 to 16 days, varying among individuals. It begins on the first day of menstrual bleeding, overlapping with the menstrual phase, and culminates in the release of a mature egg during ovulation.

At the start of this phase, the pituitary gland in the brain releases increasing amounts of follicle-stimulating hormone (FSH). FSH travels to the ovaries and stimulates the growth of multiple follicles, which each contain an immature egg. As the follicles develop, they release E2, which causes the uterine lining to thicken and become more receptive to a fertilized egg. This is known as proliferation. Though multiple follicles begin to grow, typically only one dominant follicle (with an egg inside of it) ultimately develops, while the others undergo atresia (cell death).

The increase in E2 production from the dominant follicle causes the brain to release a surge of luteinizing hormone (LH). This LH surge is what triggers ovulation to occur.

3. **Ovulation:** Ovulation is the release of a mature egg from its dominant follicle in the ovary. This occurs around the midpoint of the menstrual cycle, approximately 10 to 16 days before the start of the next period.

After the egg is released, it is captured by the fimbriae of the nearby fallopian tube. Over the next few days, the egg travels down the fallopian tube toward the uterus. The egg has the potential to be fertilized by a sperm during this time. If fertilization occurs, the fertilized egg (zygote) begins dividing as it travels to the uterus.

Some women may experience physical signs of ovulation, such as changes in cervical mucus consistency (becoming thin and stretchy, similar to egg whites), mild pelvic discomfort, or a slight increase in basal body temperature.

4. **Luteal phase:** The luteal phase typically spans from ovulation to the onset of the start menstrual period or the establishment of a pregnancy. Its duration is relatively consistent, lasting about 12 to 14 days, although individual variations can occur.

After ovulation, the ruptured dominant follicle in the ovary that contained the ovulated egg transforms into a temporary structure known as the corpus luteum, which produces high levels of P4 and E2. These hormones prepare the uterine lining for potential embryo implantation. The uterine lining becomes thickened, rich in blood vessels and nutrients. FSH and LH levels decline during the luteal phase.

The hormonal shifts that occur during the luteal phase can cause various physical and emotional symptoms, often resembling those associated with premenstrual syndrome (PMS) such as mood swings, bloating, and fatigue.

The early embryo or unfertilized egg in the fallopian tube eventually reaches the uterus during this time. If fertilization occurs, the embryo (now called a blastocyst) has the ability to implant into the uterine lining to initiate a pregnancy. If implantation occurs, the corpus luteum continues producing P4 and E2 to support the early pregnancy until the placenta takes over hormone production a few weeks later.

If fertilization and/or implantation do not occur, the corpus luteum regresses, causing P4 and E2 levels to drop. This leads to the shedding of the uterine lining, initiating a new menstrual cycle.

Conception

After sperm enter the female reproductive tract, they swim toward the mature egg in the fallopian tube while undergoing capacitation, a series of changes that make them capable of fertilizing the egg. Once they approach the egg, sperm release enzymes that penetrate the surrounding cells (corona radiata) and the egg's shell (zona pellucida). Ultimately, one sperm penetrates the egg's shell and fuses with its inner plasma membrane, triggering a reaction that prevents other sperm from entering the egg. The sperm that enters the egg then deposits its genetic material (DNA) into the egg, which initiates a series of events to occur known as oocyte activation that can result in fertilization of the egg.

A mature egg is viable for fertilization for only about twenty-four hours. Sperm, on the other hand, can survive within the female reproductive tract for several days, creating a fertile period that spans a few days around ovulation.

Within hours after fertilization, the genetic material from the sperm and egg combines to form a single-cell zygote, which undergoes rapid cell division (mitosis) as it travels down the fallopian tube toward the uterus. Roughly three days later, the early embryo should consist of about eight cells (blastomeres). By day five, the embryo (now called a blastocyst) should consist of roughly 70-100 cells. Around six to seven days after fertilization, the blastocyst reaches the uterus and prepares for implantation in the uterine lining.

Implantation

Implantation typically occurs around six to ten days after fertilization, though the exact timing can vary. Implantation involves several steps:

1. **Apposition**: the blastocyst comes into contact with the uterine lining (endometrium) and forms a temporary, loose attachment to the lining.
2. **Adhesion**: if the location suitable for implantation, the blastocyst secretes enzymes that enable it to burrow into the endometrium.
3. **Invasion**: some of the blastocyst's cells differentiate into chorionic villi—fingerlike projections that embed the embryo into the endometrium and establish a connection with the blastocyst and maternal (or gestational carrier's) blood supply, which will provide nutrients and support for the developing pregnancy.
4. **Placentation**: cells begin forming the placenta, which will nourish the developing pregnancy.

During implantation, the cells of the developing placenta release increasing amounts of human chorionic gonadotropin (hCG), a hormone that is the basis for most pregnancy tests. The presence of hCG causes the corpus luteum in the ovary to continue producing progesterone (P4) and estradiol (E2) to maintain the uterine lining and support the early pregnancy. The corpus luteum continues this hormonal support until the placenta takes over around eight to twelve weeks.

Some people may experience mild spotting or light bleeding around the time of implantation that is often mistaken for an early period. Additionally, slight cramping or discomfort may occur as the embryo burrows into the uterine lining. It is important to note that not all embryos successfully implant. Additionally, some early pregnancies may naturally fail to progress after implantation, resulting in an early miscarriage known as a biochemical pregnancy (see Chapter 10).

Female Factor Infertility

Female factor infertility (FFI) refers to conditions that prevent a female from conceiving and/or carrying a pregnancy to term. It accounts for roughly 33 percent of infertility cases. Understanding the underlying causes of FFI is crucial for accurate diagnosis, effective treatment, and compassionate support.

Endocrine Disorders and Medical Conditions

A number of hormonal disorders can impact ovulation or implantation, resulting in female factor infertility (FFI).

Ovulation is a complex process regulated by hormonal interactions between the brain, ovaries, and reproductive tract. Ovulatory dysfunction disrupts the normal process of ovulation, leading to irregular or absent menstrual cycles. Ovulatory dysfunction can present as anovulation (ovulation does not take place at all) or with oligo-ovulation (irregular ovulation leading to infrequent or sporadic periods). These abnormalities can make it difficult to estimate the right time to attempt conception in the fertile window, decrease the opportunities for fertilization, and impair the receptivity of the uterus for implantation. Diagnosing ovulatory dysfunctions typically involves menstrual cycle tracking, hormone level assessments, and ultrasound imaging. Treatment depends on the underlying cause.

These are common endocrine disorders that can disrupt fertility:

1. **Polycystic ovary syndrome (PCOS):** an endocrine disorder characterized by irregular or absent menstrual cycles, elevated levels of androgens (male hormones), clinical hyperandrogenism (e.g., facial hair or male-pattern baldness), a high anti-Müllerian hormone (AMH) level, and/or a high number of small ovarian follicles. Anovulation or oligo-ovulation are hallmarks of PCOS due to altered signaling between the brain and the ovary and altered signaling within the ovary. Approximately 8–13 percent of reproductive-age women have PCOS, making it the most prevalent endocrine disorder causing FFI. Women with PCOS are also at an increased risk of developing metabolic issues such as insulin resistance and type 2 diabetes.

    For those with PCOS, lifestyle modifications such as weight management and regular exercise can help improve hormonal balance and restore ovulation. Oral medications to induce ovulation include clomiphene citrate or letrozole, which both lead to increased FSH production by the pituitary gland. In more severe cases, gonadotropin injections might be used for ovulation induction or IVF may be recommended.

2. **Hypothalamic amenorrhea:** a condition where the brain does not produce the right amount of hormones necessary for ovulation. The hypothalamus is a region of the brain responsible for producing gonadotropin-releasing hormone (GnRH). GnRH production triggers the release of follicle-stimulating hormone (FSH) and luteinizing hormone

(LH) from the pituitary gland in the brain. GnRH is normally produced when the ovaries require FSH and LH during the follicular phase of the menstrual cycle (see section above). Hypothalamic amenorrhea disrupts the communication between the hypothalamus and ovaries, which inhibits GnRH production (and thus FSH and LH production) and causes the absence of menstrual periods and ovulation.

High amounts of emotional or physical stress (under-nutrition, excessive exercise) can lead to hypothalamic amenorrhea. While the incidence is rare, patients with hypothalamic amenorrhea should be evaluated for a brain tumor. Treating hypothalamic amenorrhea may involve addressing the underlying factors such as stress or excessive exercise and making lifestyle adjustments. If needed, injectable FSH and LH can be administered to grow one or more follicles in the ovaries. Once they have grown, medications that trigger ovulation can be administered. In refractory cases, IVF may be recommended.

Type 2 diabetes and insulin resistance: these conditions can also disrupt ovarian function and increase androgen production, leading to irregular ovulation. Uncontrolled diabetes is also associated with an increased risk of miscarriage, pregnancy complications, and birth defects.

Luteal phase defect (LPD, also called luteal phase deficiency): a condition in which the corpus luteum does not produce a normal amount of progesterone (P4), or the uterus does not respond to P4. As a result, the uterine lining does not thicken appropriately, which can hinder embryo implantation or maintenance of the early pregnancy (though healthy pregnancies are possible). While the exact cause of LPD is unknown, stress, obesity, eating disorders such as anorexia, thyroid conditions, excessive exercise, hormone imbalances such as PCOS, and endometriosis can increase the risk of LPD. Symptoms include short luteal phases (typically less than ten days), spotting or bleeding between periods, frequent or heavy periods, infertility, and early miscarriage. LPD is most commonly diagnosed through an ultrasound to measure the thickness of the uterine lining after ovulation, and a blood test to measure P4 levels during the luteal phase. Treatment options include P4 supplementation (pills, injections, or vaginal suppositories) or other medications that stimulate follicle growth or increase P4 production.

Hyperprolactinemia: a condition in which there are elevated levels of prolactin, a hormone secreted by the pituitary gland in the brain that is responsible for breast milk production. Hyperprolactinemia can suppress ovulation, leading to irregular cycles and infertility. It is most commonly diagnosed through a blood test, but important to rule out any structural abnormality in the pituitary gland when high prolactin levels are diagnosed. This usually includes a brain MRI to rule out any tumors (usually benign) that could be increasing prolactin secretion. Oral medications that stimulate dopamine receptors can suppress prolactin levels. Rarely, surgery is needed.

Abnormal thyroid function: conditions, including hypothyroidism (underactive thyroid) and hyperthyroidism (overactive thyroid), can impact ovulation, implantation, and embryo/fetal development, increasing the risk of infertility and miscarriage.

A common cause of hypothyroidism is Hashimoto's thyroiditis, an autoimmune disease in which the body's immune system mistakenly produces antibodies that attack the thyroid gland, leading to chronic inflammation and damage. Thyroid hormone supplementation can be prescribed to restore thyroid hormone levels. A common cause of hyperthyroidism is Grave's disease, an autoimmune disease that causes the thyroid to become overactive. Medications that block thyroid hormone production can optimize thyroid function. In some cases, radioactive iodine therapy or surgical removal of all or part of the thyroid may be recommended. If you take thyroid medications and become pregnant, your thyroid medication doses may need adjusted throughout your pregnancy.

Adrenal disorders: The adrenal glands are small organs that sit on top of the kidneys. There is a complex interplay between the adrenal glands, the ovaries, and the brain. The adrenal glands produce cortisol, a hormone involved in stress response and metabolism, and androgens (male sex hormones). Excess cortisol production (e.g., from chronic stress or Cushing's syndrome) and/or androgen production (e.g., from congenital adrenal hyperplasia (CAH)) can disrupt the delicate balance of hormones required for ovulation, conception, implantation, and pregnancy. Adrenal insufficiency (e.g., Addison's disease) can also affect fertility. Treatment depends on the underlying cause, but often includes medication to restore hormone levels or stress management. In some cases, fertility treatment such as IVF may also be necessary.

8. **Primary ovarian insufficiency (POI, also called premature ovarian failure):** this condition involves the loss of ovarian function before the age of forty (unlike menopause, which normally occurs around 50+ years of age). POI can result from autoimmune reactions, genetic conditions such as Fragile X or Turner syndrome, hormonal imbalances, exposure to toxins, chemotherapy, thyroid disease, or surgery on the ovaries. Those with thyroid disease, certain infections, or a family history of POI are at greater risk of developing POI. Individuals with POI often present with very low ovarian reserve (egg counts) and irregular or absent menstrual cycles, which can lead to challenges in conceiving. While there is a small chance of spontaneous conception with POI, many people require IVF, often with donor eggs or embryos, to conceive. Young women who are diagnosed with POI in adolescence, especially prior to or at the start of puberty, often need estrogen therapy to help develop the reproductive organs so they may carry a pregnancy in the future. Hormone replacement therapy is typically recommended for POI.

9. **Certain medical conditions**, such as autoimmune disorders and cancer, as well as treatments like chemotherapy and radiation, can impact ovarian function and fertility. It is important to discuss your medical history with your provider to create a personalized diagnostic and treatment plan. Collaboration with specialists who manage underlying conditions (e.g., diabetes, autoimmune diseases) is critical to ensure comprehensive care. In cases where medical treatments may compromise fertility, fertility preservation through egg or embryo freezing may be recommended prior to beginning treatment. Taking these steps can help protect future reproductive options and empower individuals to make informed decisions about their care.

Structural Abnormalities

Uterus

Uterine structural abnormalities can interfere with embryo implantation, disrupt menstrual flow, and contribute to infertility or miscarriage. Certain structural changes, including uterine fibroids, polyps, or adhesions (scar tissue), develop over time after the onset of puberty. However, structural abnormalities (Müllerian anomalies) result from abnormal uterine development during fetal growth. Examples include bicornuate uterus (a heart-shared uterus with two distinct horns), a unicornuate uterus (only half of the uterus develops), uterine didelphys (a complete double uterus with two cervixes and/or vaginas), septate uterus (a wall of tissue divides the uterine cavity), and Müllerian agenesis (MRKH syndrome, (an absent or underdeveloped uterus, cervix, and/or vagina).

Uterine fibroids (leiomyomas) are noncancerous growths that develop in or on the uterus. They are composed of muscle and connective tissue and can vary greatly in size and location. They are typically found within the uterine wall (intramural), inside the uterine cavity (submucosal), or on the outer surface of the uterus (subserosal). In some cases, fibroids can distort the uterine cavity or interfere with the shape of the uterus, which can interfere with sperm reaching the egg in the fallopian tube, hinder embryo implantation, and cause pregnancy complications. While some women with fibroids experience no symptoms, others may experience heavy or painful menstrual bleeding. Treatment depends on the location and severity of the fibroid but might bleeding. an embolization (blocking blood flow to shrink the fibroid(s)) or a myomectomy (surgical removal of the fibroid(s)).

Uterine polyps are growths of endometrial tissue that protrude into the uterine cavity. They can vary in size and location. While rare, some polyps can be or become cancerous. While many women with polyps have no symptoms, some may experience irregular or heavy periods, spotting between periods, and infertility. Polyps are typically diagnosed via imaging such as an ultrasound, sonohysterogram (SHG), or hysteroscopy. The most common treatment option is a polypectomy, or surgical removal of the polyp.

Uterine adhesions (Asherman's syndrome) are bands of scar tissue that form inside the uterus, potentially causing its walls to stick together. The adhesions are usually the result of trauma to the uterine lining from surgical procedures or severe infections (endometritis). The adhesions can decrease the amount of healthy endometrial tissue available for an embryo to attach and restrict blood flow to the uterine lining. While some women with uterine adhesions have no symptoms, others may experience light or absent periods, painful periods, infertility, or recurrent miscarriage.

Endometriosis is a chronic condition in which tissue similar to endometrial tissue forms lesions outside of the uterus, most often in the pelvis. It affects roughly 10% of reproductive-age women. This tissue behaves like endometrial tissue, thickening and breaking down during each menstrual cycle under the influence of hormones. Endometriosis can be found in the middle, muscular layer of the uterus (myometrium) in a condition known as adenomyosis. It can also attach to the ovary, forming dark, fluid-filled cysts (endometriomas or "chocolate cysts").

Endometriosis can cause pain during menstruation, intercourse, bowel movements, and urination. It can also cause bloating, heavy periods, bloating, constipation, diarrhea, and nausea. While endometriosis does not always cause infertility, it can impact fertility by interfering with ovulation, altering hormone levels, and causing pelvic inflammation. Treatment options include pain relief medications, hormone therapy, and surgery (a laparoscopy) to remove the lesions.

Fallopian Tubes

Following ovulation, an unfertilized egg is picked up by fingerlike projections (fimbriae) on the nearby fallopian tube. The egg enters the tube and travels toward the uterus for several days. During this time, fertilization can occur if sperm are present in the fallopian tube. Eventually, the egg (or embryo) enters the uterus, where implantation can occur. Blocked or damaged fallopian tubes can prevent sperm from reaching the egg or hinder the transport of the embryo to the uterus.

Infections (specifically sexually transmitted infections [STIs]), pelvic inflammatory disease (PID), inflammatory conditions of the pelvis (e.g., ruptured appendix, endometriosis, inflammatory bowel disease), or previous pelvic or abdominal surgeries can contribute to tubal scarring or damage.

A common cause of tubal factor infertility is hydrosalpinx, a condition where the fallopian tube becomes blocked and fills with fluid. This can be diagnosed via ultrasound, laparoscopy, or hysterosalpingogram (HSG). A common treatment option is a salpingostomy, during which a new opening is created in the blocked tube(s), the fluid is drained, and, in some cases, damaged portions of the tube(s) are removed. The entire affected tube can be removed via a salpingectomy. If both tubes are extensively or irreparably damaged, IVF is typically recommended to bypass the tubes. However, hydrosalpinx should be treated before an embryo transfer because its presence can reduce pregnancy rates and increase the risk of miscarriage.

Age and Reproductive Aging

Advancing age significantly affects female fertility. Women are born with a finite number of eggs (around 1–2 million at birth), and the quantity and quality of their eggs (ovarian reserve) decline over time. This decline becomes more pronounced after the age of thirty-five, leading to lower fertility rates, increased risk of miscarriage, and higher incidence of chromosomal abnormalities in eggs.

Diminished ovarian reserve (DOR) can result in irregular ovulation, making it challenging to predict fertile periods for conception and potentially disrupting hormonal support for implantation and early pregnancy. Ovarian reserve is typically assessed using blood anti-Müllerian hormone (AMH) levels or an antral follicle count (AFC), which counts the number of follicles that begin to grow at the start of a menstrual cycle.

Advancing age is also associated with a decrease in egg quality, which can impair fertilization and embryo development while also increasing the likelihood of genetic abnormalities in each embryo. Chromosomal abnormalities in embryos lead to an increased risk of miscarriage and genetic conditions such as Trisomy 21 (Down syndrome).

With advancing age also comes an increased risk for certain medical conditions. The likelihood of gynecological conditions (e.g., endometriosis, PCOS, uterine fibroids) may increase with age, potentially impacting fertility by affecting the reproductive organs. Advancing age is also often accompanied by an increased prevalence of chronic health conditions (e.g., diabetes, hypertension), which can increase the risk for infertility. These factors can further impact fertility and increase the risks of miscarriage and pregnancy complications (e.g., gestational diabetes, high blood pressure, Cesarean section, stillbirth).

While age-related decline in fertility cannot be reversed, assisted reproductive technologies such as in vitro fertilization (IVF) can help individuals conceive later in life. However, reduced egg quality and quantity may lower success rates. Egg or embryo freezing at a younger age is a proactive option for preserving fertility and improving the chances of successful conception in the future.

Unexplained Infertility

Perhaps the most frustrating diagnosis in reproductive medicine is unexplained infertility, which is given to those who are unable to conceive even after all common causes of infertility have been ruled out. In other words, all standard fertility testing has revealed no identifiable cause of infertility. Roughly 30 percent of infertile couples are diagnosed with unexplained infertility. In some cases, more advanced testing may help uncover subtle or previously undetected factors. However, it's important to know that many people with unexplained infertility are able to conceive on their own or through fertility treatment such as IVF. Your fertility specialist can help determine the best course of treatment based on your age and medical history.

Lifestyle and Environmental Factors

Lifestyle choices and environmental exposures can have a significant impact on female reproductive health and may contribute to infertility. These factors include body composition and nutrition, habits such as smoking or alcohol intake, stress and poor sleep, and environmental exposures. For more information, please see Chapter 12.

> ### Kayla's Story
>
> *When my son was three, my husband and I decided to try to have another child. After stopping my birth control and TTC for a few months, we went to my OBGYN and asked for help. She refused to test or even examine me, and told me that I just needed to keep trying and come back in a year since I had one successful pregnancy and was under thirty-five.*
>
> *After a year of no success, I returned begging for help. This time she told me to "lose weight" and "not stress about it."*
>
> *A few months later, my husband and I found a new OBGYN. This doctor sent my husband for a semen analysis, which came back as normal, and recommended that I take Clomid. However, I wasn't okay with just turning to medication when we hadn't yet discovered why I couldn't get pregnant.*
>
> *I knew there were blood or hormone tests that could be performed to determine the source of my secondary infertility. My gut told me to seek*

out a fertility specialist, which is exactly what we did, and I immediately knew that we had made the correct choice. After a fifteen-minute Zoom call, my new doctor ordered blood work that showed an elevated level of inflammation that could indicate endometriosis. I also learned that my extremely painful and heavy periods were a sign of endometriosis, which was something I had dismissed for years because I thought it was normal.

An HSG (hysterosalpingogram) was later performed to check my fallopian tubes, and then we ended up completing three IUIs with Clomid without success. We did an IVF cycle and froze four embryos, but only one embryo came back as genetically normal. I was now thirty-four and my egg supply and quality were diminishing with each passing year.

My doctor suggested that I have laparoscopic surgery performed to determine if I had endometriosis and needed additional medication to help make the embryo transfer as successful as possible. During the procedure, the doctor found and removed the tissue causing my endometriosis. Then we transferred our single embryo and it stuck! I am now over halfway through a healthy pregnancy and forever grateful for everyone at my fertility clinic helping me learn answers to my questions and get pregnant.

I learned through this whole process that we, as women, are dismissed so easily. We are given poor medical advice (such as "don't worry about it" or "try for a year"), when we, as a whole, are not educated on the female anatomy, menstruation, ovulation, etc. We have to take charge of our own health care and advocate for ourselves, and demand answers without being dismissed.

People are waiting to have children at a later age, yet there is limited information and education available about egg quality and the possible consequences of waiting to have children later in life. I wish I had sought out a fertility specialist sooner. I wish I had demanded answers sooner. I wish I had frozen my eggs in my twenties. But I just didn't think about it at that time.

Conclusions

Female factor infertility (FFI) can arise from a multitude of factors, each contributing to the complexity of the diagnosis and treatment process. A comprehensive evaluation, including medical history, physical examination, hormonal assessments, and imaging studies can help to determine the underlying cause of infertility.

With advances in reproductive medicine and assisted reproductive technologies, many individuals facing infertility can explore treatment options tailored to their specific needs and circumstances. An individualized and multidisciplinary approach is imperative. Understanding the causes, impact, and available treatments for FFI empowers both medical professionals and individuals to work collaboratively toward family building and optimizing reproductive health.

Chapter 4
Meeting Your Fertility Specialist

The following information was submitted by Mark Surrey, MD, FACOG, FACS, co-founder of SCRC.

Finding a fertility specialist is an important step in many fertility journeys. These medical professionals help individuals and couples facing challenges with conception or carrying a pregnancy to term. The most common type of fertility specialist is a Reproductive Endocrinologist and Infertility (REI) specialist, a gynecologist with advanced training in reproductive medicine. Urologists with fellowships in male fertility also play a critical role in addressing male factor infertility. Fertility specialists often work with a multidisciplinary team that may include physician assistants, nurses, embryologists, andrologists, sonographers, and medical assistants. Additional support can include acupuncturists, mental health specialists, and nutritionists.

When to See a Fertility Specialist

You should consider seeing a fertility specialist if you:

- Are struggling to conceive or maintain a pregnancy
- Have questions about your reproductive health
- Have a diagnosed or suspected reproductive disorder
- Are interested in preserving your fertility for the future

- Require third-party reproductive options (e.g., donor eggs or sperm)
- Have concerns about passing on a genetic condition to your children

Preparing for your Appointment

Your first appointment with a fertility specialist can naturally come with a range of emotions. Many people feel nervous, confused, intimidated, stressed, or anxious prior to the appointment. These emotions are all normal considering that fertility is such a deeply personal topic, and decisions such as preserving your fertility or wanting children do not come lightly.

Before your appointment, educate yourself about fertility and treatment options (this guide is a great resource!). Coming in armed with knowledge will help you feel more confident. Additionally, you (and your partner, if applicable) can best prepare for your first appointment by:

- Writing down your personal fertility goals and objectives. For example:
  - Do you desire to have one child or multiple children? How long do you wish to wait between births?
  - Are you willing to undergo IVF if needed? How many cycles are you willing to complete?
- Compiling a list of specific questions regarding your fertility or treatment options. For example:
  - Which treatments does the clinic offer?
    - Note: if IVF is not included in the list of treatments, consider finding a clinic that offers IVF. If the clinic does offer IVF, be sure to ask how many cycles a year the clinic performs and what its clinical pregnancy rate is **in pertinence to your age range and condition**.
  - What are the clinic's success rates compared to national averages?
  - What diagnostic tests will you need to complete before you begin treatment?
  - What is your recommended treatment option and why?
  - Is there a waitlist for treatment at the clinic? If so, how long will it take before you can begin treatment?
  - What does the timeline look like for the treatment that is recommended?

- Should you be taking any vitamins or supplements to optimize your chances of success?
- What should you be doing to optimize your chance of success? What should you avoid?
- If IUI cycles are recommended, how many cycles should you complete before moving to IVF?
- How can you get in touch with someone at the clinic during and after business hours?
- Does the clinic offer payment plans, financing options, payment packages, or grants? What are the estimated costs?
- How many treatment cycles might you need based on your fertility goals and diagnosis?
- Does the clinic offer any mental health resources or have a recommended mental health specialist who focuses on infertility?
- What are your next steps following this appointment?

- Creating a list of important future event dates (vacations, weddings) that may interfere with your treatment. This can help you plan when to begin your treatment cycles.
- Sending any relevant medical records (both yours and your partner's, if applicable) to the clinic so your fertility specialist can review these records prior to your visit. It helps to keep copies of these records for yourself, as well.
  - If you feel comfortable doing so, gather relevant medical information from your family members. This includes any history of fertility issues, pregnancy losses, reproductive abnormalities, and known genetic conditions within your family.
  - It may help to make a quick reference list of your fertility history. This might include the date of your last menstrual period, the age you began having menstrual cycles, the date of your last gynecologist visit, any relevant test results, and your current list of medications.
- Completing pre-visit intake forms from the clinic. These are often sent electronically, though some clinics also utilize paper intake forms.

- Doing your research on your clinic and fertility specialist so you feel more comfortable prior to arriving. This information can typically be found on the clinic's website and may include your specialist's biography as well as your clinic's treatment options and success rates.
- Checking to see if your health insurance covers any costs associated with fertility treatment at your clinic.

On the day of your appointment, you should arrive at least fifteen minutes prior to your appointment time (unless instructed otherwise) so you are not rushed in the event of unexpected delays. You should bring:

- Your health insurance card(s)
- A government-issued ID (e.g., driver's license or passport) for yourself and your partner (if applicable)
- Any other documentation that your clinic requires for this appointment
- A notebook or an electronic device to take notes
- A method of payment (e.g., credit card)

Most clinics have a reception area where you can check in and fill out any additional forms before your appointment begins.

The Initial Consultation

During your first appointment with a fertility specialist, you can expect to:

- Discuss your medical and reproductive history, including any concerns, questions, and personal goals related to your fertility.
- Complete a pelvic ultrasound to assess your reproductive anatomy.
- Have your blood drawn to evaluate your hormone levels. Additional blood tests and/or a physical exam may also be necessary depending on certain factors. For example, if a male partner is present, he may need to provide a semen sample so a semen analysis can be performed.
- Schedule additional testing (if needed) or your next appointment or procedure.

Don't hesitate to speak up and ask questions! If you don't understand something, ask for clarification. Fertility specialists and their teams are there to support you—they want to help you reach your goals and are committed to providing expert, compassionate care.

Receiving Your Diagnosis and Treatment Plan

After your initial consultation, your fertility specialist will review the results of your ultrasound, bloodwork, and any other tests that were performed at the appointment. While some individuals receive a diagnosis based on this initial round of testing, others require additional diagnostic testing to receive a diagnosis. Please see Chapter 5 for more information about diagnostic testing options.

After you receive your diagnosis, you and your fertility specialist can develop a personalized treatment plan. You will receive your instructions based on the results of this conversation.

Important Considerations

It is important to remember that the outcome of your fertility journey may very well be determined by the quality of care you receive. This is why it is important to be discerning when selecting a fertility specialist. This decision can shape your path forward. Don't be nervous, but be prepared and informed in your selection! Interview your specialist to ensure they have the correct experience, expertise, and treatment offerings that align with your specific fertility needs. Look for someone with a proven track record of helping individuals with similar diagnoses and goals. With the right fertility specialist, you should feel that you are in expert hands and supported every step of the way. If you do not feel that you are receiving the level of care you deserve, it's okay to seek a second (or third) opinion until you feel confident in your decision to move forward with a fertility specialist.

> ### *Baby S's Story*
>
> *My husband and I were trying to conceive for about eight months, but I knew that something was off when I started tracking my ovulation. We began treatment with timed intercourse for three cycles and then intrauterine insemination (IUI) for another three cycles. All of these cycles failed. To top it off, I was forgotten about in my exam room while waiting for my final IUI. I could even hear the nurses going back and forth outside of my door for two whole hours.*
>
> *And that was enough. We left the clinic forever.*
>
> *My husband and I tried to naturally conceive while taking a break from treatment for a year and a half. Finally, we got into a new clinic and, for the first time ever, got a diagnosis. It turns out that I have stage 4 endometriosis, which didn't surprise me at all!*
>
> *We were able to conceive with our first IUI at the new clinic, but unfortunately the pregnancy was ectopic. After waiting for three months, we finally began IVF treatment and ended up with seven embryos that have passed genetic testing and are frozen!*
>
> *My advice is to advocate for yourself and don't stop looking until you find the right clinic. And don't forget to take time for yourself and lean on your support system. I used to be in complete fear of going through IVF and never thought I could go through with it. But by taking things at my own pace and finding my support system, I can honestly say that I'm looking forward to my transfer!*

Conclusions

Feeling comfortable and confident in your fertility clinic and specialist is essential. You're investing significant time, energy, and resources into your care team, so it's important to be prepared, ask questions, and advocate for yourself every step of the way. The right specialist will not only offer expertise but also make you feel supported, respected, and heard throughout your journey.

Chapter 5

Diagnostic Tests and Treatment Options

The following information was submitted by Phoebe Howells, BSc(Hons), MBBch, MRCOG. A senior registrar in obstetrics and gynecology and chief medical officer for OVUM.

If you've just completed your first consultation with a fertility specialist, you may be feeling a whirlwind of emotions-hope and anticipation as you move one step closer to your dream, anxiety from the amount of information you had to absorb in a short amount of time, and nervousness about your next steps. These feelings are completely normal. And yes, they often lead to a flurry of internet searches. This chapter will break down the most common diagnostic tests used to investigate your cause of infertility, along with the various treatment options your fertility specialist may recommend for you based on your diagnosis.

Investigating Your Cause of Infertility

There are many diagnostic tests that can help determine your underlying cause of infertility. Some of these tests may be performed during your initial consultation, while others are performed at a later date. Some individuals require multiple diagnostic tests, while others will discover their cause of infertility more rapidly. This section outlines some common tests that can be performed in a basic fertility workup, but you likely won't need to complete all of them. Advanced testing may be recommended based on your medical history and/or the results of your initial tests.

Blood tests

1. **Anti-Müllerian hormone (AMH) level.** AMH is produced by granulosa cells, which eggs inside their follicles within the ovaries. It plays a key role in the regulation of ovarian function, particularly in the development and maturation of eggs (oocytes).

    AMH levels are typically measured to assess the quantity of eggs remaining in the ovaries (ovarian reserve). In general, a high AMH level indicates a higher higher ovarian reserve, while a low AMH level indicates the opposite. Higher AMH levels can be associated with conditions such as polycystic ovary syndrome PCOS, while lower levels can be associated with diminished ovarian reserve (DOR) or primary ovarian insufficiency (POI). Your AMH level can help determine when you should begin fertility treatment, which treatment options and medication dosages are best for you, and how your ovaries might respond to stimulation medications. It's important to remember that AMH levels alone cannot definitively predict your fertility or provide information about the quality of your eggs.

    There are many factors that can affect AMH levels, though the main factor is age. In general, ovarian reserve and AMH levels decline with age.

2. **Infectious disease screening.** Infectious diseases can be transmitted between partners and from a pregnant person to the developing fetus. Certain infections can pose significant risks during pregnancy to the mother/carrier and fetus. Identifying and managing these infections can help prevent disease transmission and complications during fertility treatment and pregnancy. It is also important to know these results to prevent transmission of diseases to the clinic staff, as well as from donor eggs/sperm to the recipient(s). Before you begin fertility treatment, you may be asked to complete infectious disease screening, which typically includes testing for:

    – HIV
    – Hepatitis B (HBV)

- Hepatitis C (HCV)
- Cytomegalovirus (if applicable)
- Syphilis (RPR)

3. **Immunity screening.** These tests determine if you are immune to Rubella (German Measles) and Varicella (Chickenpox), viruses that can cause severe birth defects if acquired during pregnancy. For those who are non-immune to these infections, vaccination is recommended and efforts are made to ensure that pregnancy is not pursued until immunity is confirmed.

4. **Thyroid hormone testing.** Up to 5 percent of women struggling to conceive have abnormal thyroid hormone levels, which can interfere with conception and cause pregnancy complications if left untreated (see Chapter 3). Therefore, thyroid levels should be within normal ranges prior to conception or the start of fertility treatment.

    The primary thyroid hormone that is measured is thyroid-stimulating hormone (TSH). High TSH levels suggest an underactive thyroid (hypothyroidism), while low TSH levels suggest an overactive thyroid (hyperthyroidism). Your clinic may also measure your Free T4 (FT4) or Free T3 (FT3) levels and test for thyroid antibodies such as thyroid peroxidase antibodies (TPO-Ab), depending on your medical history.

5. **Reproductive hormone testing.** You and your partner (if applicable) may be asked to have any or all of the following blood tests to check your hormone levels to determine if there are any underlying causes of infertility.

    For females:

- Follicle-stimulating hormone (FSH) stimulates the growth of the follicles that contain the eggs inside of your ovaries. The test should be taken around day 3 of your menstrual cycle (your cycle begins on the first day of menses) for accurate interpretation. If you are not having periods, it may be because this hormone is very low. High levels can indicate low ovarian reserve or primary ovarian insufficiency (POI).
- Luteinizing hormone (LH) stimulates the rapid growth of the dominant follicle (the follicle that the egg will ovulate from) and triggers ovulation to occur. It is often tested around day 3 of the menstrual cycle. If you are not ovulating, your LH levels can help determine the cause. For example, a high LH level may suggest PCOS, though consistently high levels can also suggest menopause. Low levels

can prevent ovulation from occurring. Extreme exercise, high stress, eating disorders, or disorders of the pituitary gland in the brain can cause low LH levels. Women with low day-3 LH levels are less likely to respond well to ovarian stimulation medications used in fertility treatment such as IVF.
- Estradiol (E2) is secreted by ovarian follicles and should be measured around day 3 of the menstrual cycle. A high E2 can indicate a diminished ovarian reserve (DOR), especially with a normal FSH level.
- Prolactin levels can be checked at any point in the menstrual cycle. Levels vary throughout the day and are highest when you are asleep and first thing in the morning, so the test is usually done three hours after you wake up. High prolactin levels can prevent your brain from secreting FSH, which can prevent eggs from maturing and ovulation from occurring. Levels can be high due to medication use (some antidepressants and painkillers), hypothyroidism, stress, lack of sleep, or, in rare cases, a pituitary tumor. Therefore, you may be asked to have an MRI scan to exclude any such tumors. Reversing these causes may improve the regularity of your menstrual cycles and therefore improve your fertility.

For males:

- Testosterone is the primary male sex hormone, and low levels can have a direct impact on male fertility by impacting sperm production. Levels tend to drop as men age. Testosterone levels can be checked at any time but are highest in the morning.
- Follicle-stimulating hormone (FSH) stimulates the production of sperm in the testes. High levels can indicate testicular damage or failure, while low levels can indicate issues with the hypothalamus or pituitary gland in the brain. Testing is usually recommended for men who have a reduced total motile sperm count.
- Luteinizing hormone (LH) works with FSH to stimulate the production of testosterone in the testes. Low LH levels are typically associated with low testosterone levels, which can result in reduced sperm production. Abnormal levels can be a result of testicular damage or issues with the hypothalamus or pituitary gland in the brain.
- Prolactin levels may be measured in cases of low testosterone since high prolactin levels can cause abnormal sperm production, low testosterone levels, and infertility.

Diagnostic procedures

1. **Fertility assessment scan (FAS) or pelvic exam.** The name of this scan may vary between clinics, but it typically involves a transvaginal ultrasound scan (TVUS), in which a long, thin probe (often nicknamed "Wanda") with a plastic cover is inserted into the vagina. TVUS images of the ovaries and uterus are much clearer versus a transabdominal (on the stomach) ultrasound, but a transabdominal ultrasound can be used for those who have difficulty with penetration or have not had intercourse.

    This assessment will look for any abnormalities or clues as to why you are having difficulty conceiving. It often assesses:

    – The size and shape of your uterus, thickness of your uterine lining (endometrium), and presence of any abnormalities such as fibroids or polyps (see Chapter 3).
    – The size and shape of your ovaries.
    – Your antral follicle count (AFC), which measures the number of small follicles in your ovaries at the beginning of your menstrual cycle. Your AFC is used in conjunction with your AMH level (described above) to predict your ovarian reserve and response to fertility stimulation medications. AFCs can vary from cycle to cycle.

2. **Saline infusion sonogram (SIS) or sonohysterogram (SHG).** This procedure evaluates your uterine cavity in greater detail than a standard ultrasound. It helps detect polyps, fibroids, scar tissue, or other uterine abnormalities that may impact fertility.

    Before the procedure, you may receive guidance to take an over-the-counter pain relief medication since the procedure can cause abdominal cramping. During the procedure, a small catheter is inserted through your cervix and into your uterus. Once the catheter is in position, a small amount of saline solution is introduced into your uterus to expand the cavity. The cavity is visualized using an abdominal ultrasound, and any protrusions or irregularities should become visible during this process. Afterward, you and your fertility specialist can determine whether it is necessary to remove these growths.

    This procedure is minimally invasive and usually takes around ten minutes to complete. It's recommended that you bring someone with you so they can drive you home if you experience pain afterward. While some people experience minimal pain, others may find that it makes them feel faint and dizzy, and occasionally people can pass out. This is due to the manipulation of the cervix during the procedure, which can cause a temporary fall in blood pressure (cervical shock).

The procedure carries a small risk of infection, so a prophylactic antibiotic is often prescribed on the day of the procedure. Let your care team know if you feel unwell in the days or weeks following the procedure and experience fever, loss of appetite, or abnormal vaginal discharge.

Occasionally, the catheter cannot be passed through the cervix far enough to remain in place. There are different catheters that can be used to overcome this, but occasionally it is not possible to gain entry into the cavity and the procedure cannot be completed. This may be the case in those who have had prior cervical treatments.

3. **Hysterosalpingo-contrast sonography (HyCoSy).** This procedure assesses the uterine cavity and patency (openness) of the fallopian tubes. Various factors, such as a history of STIs, past abdominal surgeries, and endometriosis, can lead to inflammation and scarring, which cause adhesions that block the tubes. The HyCoSy procedure is sometimes recommended before beginning ovulation induction or intrauterine insemination (IUI) to determine if the tubes are open. If they are not, these treatment options will not be effective.

A HyCoSy can be performed with a SIS/SHG, utilizing the same catheter inserted through the cervix. During this procedure, a contrast medium is injected into the uterus and visualized via transvaginal ultrasound. If the tubes are open, the contrast medium will flow freely through them.

However, if the contrast medium encounters an obstruction and does not pass through the tubes, it may suggest either a genuine blockage or temporary spasm of the tube, which causes it to clamp down while the contrast medium passes through. In either case, you will have the opportunity to decide the next steps, which may include a repeat HyCoSy, in vitro fertilization (IVF), or further exploration through a laparoscopy with dye (see below).

A HyCoSy takes around fifteen minutes to complete, and your doctor might recommend that you take pain medication before the procedure since many people find this procedure uncomfortable and painful. It is best to bring someone with you to escort you home.

A HyCoSy carries the same risks as the SIS/SHG. Neither of these procedures can be performed if there is any chance of pregnancy, so you may be told to abstain from sexual intercourse from the beginning of your period until the test. They also cannot be performed if you are suspected to have a pelvic infection or a history of hydrosalpinx (fluid in the tube), as these procedures could make the infection worse.

4. **Hysterosalpingography (HSG)**. Though HSG and HyCOSy procedures are similar, some clinics may offer one instead of the other. An HSG also determines if there is a blockage in the fallopian tubes and is therefore indicated for patients who have a history of STIs, previous abdominal surgeries, endometriosis, or for those undergoing ovulation induction or IUI. It can also assess the uterine cavity, which helps identify abnormalities such as polyps, fibroids, scar tissue, or congenital abnormalities (structural issues present at birth). However, HSGs tend to provide a less detailed view of the uterine cavity compared to an SIS/SHG or HyCoSy.

   An HSG involves injecting a contrast dye into the uterus and fallopian tubes. An X-ray is then used to evaluate the uterus and patency of the fallopian tubes. The timing can vary, but it generally takes about fifteen to thirty minutes to complete. Pain medication is recommended before this procedure since it can cause discomfort and pain. It is best to bring someone with you to escort you home.

5. **Hysteroscopy.** This procedure can be both diagnostic and surgical. It involves the use of a hysteroscope (a slender, lighted tube with a camera), which is gently inserted through the cervix into the uterine cavity. Saline solution or gas is injected to expand the uterus , allowing for the direct visualization of the uterine cavity and openings to the fallopian tubes to detect any abnormalities (e.g., polyps, fibroids).

   If previous image testing revealed the presence of a polyp, a fibroid, a septum, or scar tissue in the uterus, it may be necessary to undergo a hysteroscopy for treatment to remove the abnormality, though treatment is not always necessary. Treatment involves inserting small instruments through the hysteroscope to surgically remove the abnormalities.

   The hysteroscopy procedure can be performed on an outpatient basis with local or no anesthesia while you are awake, or under general anesthesia while you are asleep. Your specialist will help determine which option is best for you. Regardless, someone should be available to drive you home following the procedure.

6. **Laparoscopy and dye test.** This minimally invasive procedure is considered the gold standard for assessing fallopian tube

patency (openness), diagnosing and evaluating pelvic anatomy. It is recommended if you have a history of abdominal surgery or inconclusive results from a HyCoSy or HSG.

A laparoscopy with dye is performed under general anesthesia. During the procedure, your abdomen is filled with carbon dioxide gas to create space. This enables the insertion of a camera through a small incision near your navel. During this procedure, any pelvic endometriosis can be observed and adhesions can be removed as needed. Additionally, a blue dye is injected through a catheter placed in your cervix. The camera inside your abdomen allows the specialist to observe whether the dye flows through the fallopian tubes and spills out their ends. Failure of the dye to spill out indicates a blockage in the tube. The specialist can attempt to reopen the blocked tube during this procedure.

It's important to note that while this test is highly accurate, it may involve a longer waiting period due to the need to be placed on a surgical waiting list. Additionally, it carries some additional risks, so it's essential to have a thorough discussion with your fertility specialist to assess the suitability of this procedure for your specific situation and to weigh the potential benefits against the risks.

7. **Endometrial biopsy.** This procedure involves inserting a thin tube through the cervix into the uterus. The end of the tube scrapes the uterine lining (endometrium) to remove a small tissue sample. The biopsied sample is then sent for testing, and it can take a few weeks to get the results.

Endometrial biopsies are usually taken during the luteal (post-ovulation) phase. Specialized tests can examine the biopsied sample to determine the optimal timing for your embryo transfer based when your endometrium is most receptive to implantation, evaluate your uterine microbiome (bacteria in the uterus), and diagnose chronic endometritis (inflammation of the uterine lining). If endometritis is found, antibiotics are often recommended as a treatment option.

The procedure can cause some discomfort similar to menstrual cramping. It is important to discuss the risks and benefits of the procedure with your fertility specialist to see if this test is right for you.

Other diagnostic tests:

1. **Semen analysis or seminal fluid analysis (SFA)** As its name implies, this test analyzes a semen sample to assess male fertility.

    A semen sample can be collected either at your clinic or home (depending on your clinic's policy). A trained staff member (typically an andrologist) will use a microscope or other specialized device to analyze the sample and report the outcomes.

    Important factors include the concentration, motility, and morphology of the sperm in the sample (see Chapter 2).

2. **Genetic carrier screening.** This test, which typically consists of either a blood draw or cheek swab, can help determine your risk of passing on certain inherited genetic conditions (e.g., cystic fibrosis) to your offspring. Genetic conditions result from mutations in our genes (DNA).

    Genes come in pairs, with one copy inherited from each parent. Most genetic conditions are inherited in an autosomal recessive manner. This means that a person needs to inherit two mutated copies of the gene (one from each parent) to be affected by the condition.

    A person who is a carrier for a genetic condition has one working copy of a gene and one nonworking (mutated) copy. Carriers typically do not experience symptoms of the condition because the unaffected gene usually compensates for the mutated one.

    In fact, did you know that most people are carriers of at least one genetic condition and don't even know it? Normally, this isn't an issue. However, when two carriers of the same genetic mutation (who may not even know they're carriers) have a child, there's a 25% chance with each pregnancy that the child will be affected by the condition, a 50% chance that the child will be a carrier, and a 25% chance that the child will be neither affected nor a carrier. An autosomal recessive gene can be passed through generations without ever being known about and may only come to light when that person conceives with someone with the same mutation and their child is affected.

    At the time of your initial consultation, you might be asked about your ethnic background and family history. There are certain genetic conditions that are more prevalent in specific ethnic backgrounds and other conditions that will need to be tested for if a family member has been affected. Some fertility clinics have genetic counselors to help determine what testing is needed.

Some clinics offer expanded carrier screening, which screens for hundreds of genes simultaneously, while others offer targeted screening that focuses on a smaller panel, often for life-threatening conditions. In situations where there is a risk of a child inheriting a genetic condition, IVF with preimplantation genetic testing for monogenic disorders (PGT-M) can help identify which embryos are affected by, carriers of, or unaffected by the genetic condition before they're transferred into the uterus.

3. **Chlamydia and gonorrhea screening.** These common STIs can cause pelvic inflammatory disease (PID). If left untreated, PID can damage the fallopian tubes and other reproductive organs, resulting in tubal factor infertility (see Chapter 3) and an increased risk of ectopic pregnancy. Infection during pregnancy can lead to complications such as preterm birth, low birth weight, neonatal conjunctivitis, and pneumonia. Chlamydia and gonorrhea infections are often asymptomatic, so many people are unaware that they are infected. Testing is typically performed via a genital swab. Routine testing helps identify asymptomatic infections, allowing for timely treatment with antibiotics and preventing the development of complications that could impact fertility.

4. **Karyotype.** This test examines the number and structure of the chromosomes in your cells. They can help identify chromosomal abnormalities (e.g., translocations or inversions) that can contribute to infertility or recurrent miscarriage. In cases where structural abnormalities are found within the chromosomes, IVF with preimplantation genetic testing for structural rearrangements (PGT-SR) can be performed to identify embryos without structural rearrangements before they're transferred into the uterus. Karyotypes are typically performed on both partners via a blood test.

> ### *Giselle's Story*
>
> *My husband and I were planning to try to conceive but had some concerns about the possibility of our children being affected by fragile X syndrome since my mother's side of the family all experienced early menopause and infertility. We decided to complete genetic carrier screening and learned that, while I do not carry the fragile X genetic mutation, I am a genetic carrier for Pompe disease. My husband also underwent carrier screening to be cautious, and it turned out that he is also a carrier for Pompe disease. We then had to make the difficult decision to determine if IVF was the best option to prevent having a child affected by our genetic mutations.*
>
> *We thankfully had a wonderful reproductive endocrinology department and a great doctor to help us through the process. We did our first egg retrieval in December of 2022 and ended up with seven euploid blastocysts! We went ahead with PGT-M (preimplantation genetic testing for a monogenic disease) and found that one embryo was affected with Pompe disease, two were non-carriers of the disease, and four were carriers of the disease. We were able to transfer one of our non-carriers, a 3BB, in May 2023.*
>
> *I hope that my story can show the importance of genetic carrier testing and knowing if you carry any genetic disorders. I believe that knowledge is power and can help you make the right decision for your family. My testing has allowed my sister to complete genetic carrier screening, and I have encouraged my cousins to look into it as well so they can have an awareness about what they might carry.*
>
> *I also think it's important to highlight our ability to make sure we don't pass on genetic conditions to our offspring. When talking to others, I learned that many people do not know that this is an option, so I enjoy being able to tell my story and how IVF was a part of building our family.*

Fertility Treatment Options

Note: In order to understand the different treatment protocols you must be familiar with the menstrual cycle. Please refer to Chapter 3 for more information about this.

Many people who are seen in fertility clinics do not need to go straight to IVF treatment. In fact, there are a range of treatment options that may be available depending on your diagnosis and medical history. Your fertility specialist will help determine the best approach and should be able to share your clinic's success rates for each treatment option.

1. **Natural cycle tracking and timed intercourse.** Conception can sometimes occur by tracking ovulation and performing timed intercourse (TIC) around this time. As a reminder, ovulation is the process near the middle of your menstrual cycle in which a mature egg is released from the ovary.

    There are several methods to track ovulation:

    - **Basal body temperature (BBT):** There is a noticeable rise in BBT following ovulation due to increased progesterone (P4) levels. It's best to check your BBT around the same time every morning as soon as you wake up with a specialized thermometer.
    - **Ovulation predictor kits (OPKs): These** measure the level of luteinizing hormone (LH) in your urine. A surge in LH levels usually occurs twenty-four to forty-eight hours before ovulation. To determine when to start testing calculate how many days your menstrual cycles last, subtract fourteen, and start using them a few days before that. For example, in a 28-day cycle, you would want to start testing around day 10. Some fertility clinics advise testing twice a day (twelve hours apart).
    - **Cervical mucus changes:** As you approach ovulation, your cervical mucus becomes more abundant, clearer, and more stretchy (like the consistency of raw egg whites). This is fertile cervical mucus that helps the sperm travel to the egg.
    - **Mittelschmerz:** is a one-sided, lower pelvic pain that may occur around the time of ovulation.

    Another option is to have ultrasound scans during your cycle to see when a dominant follicle (the large follicle that contains the egg which will be ovulated that cycle) arises in your ovary, and then have TIC leading up to expected ovulation and after. Exact advice on timings of intercourse will be personalized to you depending on your scan/blood findings and specified by your specialist. Sperm can survive for several days within the female genital tract, with fertilization being possible up to 5 days after entering the tract.

    There is also the option of having a trigger injection (a medication that triggers ovulation to occur) to help determine when you should have TIC. This technique alone may be all you need if you are having difficulty tracking your ovulation but have no underlying causes of infertility.

2. **Ovulation induction (OI).** Some people's menstrual cycles are very irregular, so they need to induce ovulation with the help of medications like Clomid or Letrozole. These medications move make the ovaries more responsive to FSH and LH, thereby promoting the growth of one or more follicles. Once you've responded to these medications (typically around day 10 of your cycle), you can begin monitoring your follicle(s) as they continue to grow via a transvaginal ultrasound.

    It's important to note that sometimes more than one follicle becomes dominant, meaning it grows larger than the others. In such cases, both eggs within these dominant follicles can ovulate and potentially be fertilized. This increases the possibility of having a multiple pregnancy (i.e., twins or triplets). Your fertility specialist will discuss the risks associated with multiple pregnancies and may consider canceling the cycle if more than two dominant follicles are detected due to the significant risks associated with high-order multiple pregnancies.

    Once you have identified your dominant follicle(s), you and your doctor can discuss your choices:

    - You can allow ovulation to occur naturally and track it (as discussed above), followed by TIC at home.
    - You can opt for a trigger injection when the lining of the uterus is sufficiently thick and the dominant follicle(s) has reached the desired size. You can then decide whether to proceed with intrauterine insemination (IUI) or continue with TIC at home.

3. **Intrauterine insemination (IUI).** As its name implies, intrauterine insemination refers to the injection of sperm into the uterus around the time of ovulation. IUIs can be performed using fresh or frozen sperm produced by your partner or a donor (known or unknown). Before the procedure, the sperm sample is cleaned and placed into a sterile labeled tube. During the procedure, you will lie on an exam table with your legs in stirrups and a small catheter specifically designed for this procedure will be inserted through the cervix into the uterus. The cleaned sperm is then injected into the uterus through this catheter. At this point, the sperm can swim toward the egg(s) in the fallopian tube.

IUI success rates vary between individuals and clinics. On average, the success rate per IUI cycle is roughly 10–20 percent, but this rate declines with age and depends on multiple factors such as diagnosis, medical history, and sperm quality.

Intracervical Insemination (ICI) is another form of artificial insemination used to help individuals or couples conceive. However, sperm are deposited into the vagina, close to the cervix, instead of into the uterus as with IUI. This allows the sperm to naturally migrate through the cervix into the uterus and fallopian tube to reach the egg. ICI can be performed with either unwashed (ICI-ready) or washed (IUI-ready) sperm from either a partner or donor (donor sperm banks can even ship vials of donor sperm to your house for this). ICI can often be performed at home by the individual or a partner, though some clinics may also offer ICI as a treatment option. ICI may be a suitable starting point for individuals or couples without known fertility issues, especially those using donor sperm who prefer home insemination.

4. **In vitro fertilization (IVF).** After consulting with your healthcare team, the decision to move forward with IVF may be made. However, there are still important choices to be considered as there exists a variety of protocols, each requiring customization to best suit your specific needs. The primary goal is to optimize the number of eggs retrieved while ensuring your well-being remains a top priority throughout the entire cycle. For more information about the steps involved in an IVF cycle, please see Chapter 7.

Conclusions

There are multiple diagnostic tests available to determine your cause of infertility. There are also multiple treatment options available that can help overcome infertility depending on its cause.

Chapter 6
Fertility Medications and IVF Monitoring

The information in this chapter was provided by Natasha Stamper, PharmD, a clinical pharmacist and creator of fertility pharmacist LLC.

Fertility medications play a vital role in many treatment plans. In general, these medications temporarily alter your body's natural hormonal processes to optimize your fertility outcomes. Your fertility specialist will prescribe medications based on your diagnosis (see Chapters 2 and 3), treatment plan (see Chapter 5), and medical history.

Common fertility medications include:

- **Clomiphene citrate (Clomid, Serophene)**: This oral medication is often used to treat ovulation disorders such as polycystic ovary syndrome (PCOS), anovulation (absent ovulation), unexplained infertility, and luteal phase defect. It blocks estrogen receptors in the brain, which stimulates the brain to release increasing amounts of follicle-stimulating hormone (FSH) and luteinizing hormone (LH). This increased hormonal stimulation promotes the growth and development of ovarian follicles, which contain the eggs. It is usually taken at the beginning of the menstrual cycle for five days, but this will be determined by your fertility specialist. You may complete ultrasounds and blood work during this time to track your response to the medication. Ovulation typically occurs 5-10 days after the last pill is taken, but a trigger shot is sometimes administered to induce final egg maturation and ovulation. Timed intercourse (TIC) or an intrauterine insemination (IUI) should occur around the time of ovulation as determined by your fertility specialist.

- **Aromatase inhibitors (Letrozole, Femara)**: These oral medications are sometimes used as an alternative to clomiphene citrate for inducing ovulation, especially for individuals with PCOS. These medications block estrogen production, which stimulates the brain to produce FSH and LH. This, in turn, prompts follicle development and ovulation. In males, these medications can increase testosterone levels and decrease estrogen levels, which can improve sperm production. Aromatase inhibitors typically follow the same regiment as clomiphene citrate, with or without a trigger shot, followed by TIC or an IUI.
- **Gonadotropins (Follistim, Gonal-F, Menopur)**: These injectable medications consist of follicle-stimulating hormone (FSH) and/or luteinizing hormone (LH). They directly stimulate the development of one or more follicles in the ovaries and can also be utilized in men to stimulate testosterone and sperm production. Gonadotropins are typically used during IVF, but they may be prescribed for ovulation induction with TIC or IUI when oral medications are ineffective.
- **Human chorionic gonadotropin (hCG)**: This injectable hormone is frequently used alongside other fertility medications to induce ovulation. It is similar to LH, so injecting hCG mimics the LH surge and triggers the final maturation of an egg(s) and ovulation. It can also stimulate testosterone and sperm production.
- **Metformin**: This oral medication is primarily used to treat insulin resistance and improve ovulation in individuals with PCOS.
- **Bromocriptine or Cabergoline**: These oral medications help treat high levels of prolactin (hyperprolactinemia), a hormone that can impair follicular development and prevent the dominant follicle from reaching maturation, resulting in a lack of ovulation.

Medications for In Vitro Fertilization (IVF)

IVF medications are administered in order to:

- **Stimulate the ovaries**. Normally, only one egg fully matures per menstrual cycle, which is the egg that is ovulated that cycle. IVF stimulation medications causes multiple eggs to mature simultaneously, increasing the number available for IVF.

- **Control the timing of ovulation.** Without intervention, the maturation of multiple eggs would trigger ovulation to occur, but IVF medications prevent premature ovulation, ensuring eggs remain in the ovaries until the scheduled retrieval. If ovulation occurs too early, the eggs cannot be retrieved.
- **Trigger final egg maturation.** Once the follicles have developed sufficiently, trigger medications promote the final maturation of the eggs, preparing them for retrieval and fertilization.
- **Prepare the uterine lining (endometrium) for implantation.** A thick, nutrient-rich endometrium is essential for embryo implantation and early pregnancy support. Specific medications help build and maintain this environment when an embryo transfer occurs.

IVF Medication Classes

Various medications may be used during the IVF stimulation phase. Your stimulation protocol, including the specific dosage, duration, and frequency of each medication, is determined by your fertility specialist and may be adjusted throughout the treatment cycle based on your response to the medications and desired outcome. The classes of IVF medications consist of:

1. **Gonadotropins** (menotropins (hMG, Menopur), follitropin alfa (Gonal-f), and follitropin beta (Follistim AQ)) are subcutaneous injectable hormones that consist of luteinizing hormone (LH) and/or follicle-stimulating hormone (FSH), which are normally produced by the pituitary gland in the brain. They help to stimulate the maturation of multiple eggs in the ovaries.

    Gonadotropins administration normally begins around the third day of the menstrual cycle in which IVF will occur (the first day of the menstrual cycle is cycle day 1) and continues for approximately 8–12 days, though timing may vary.

2. **Gonadotropin-releasing hormone (GnRH) agonists** (Synarel (nasal spray), Lupron, Zoladex (injections)) initially cause the brain to produce FSH and LH to stimulate follicle development. However, after a few days, they cause the brain to stop producing these hormones, which prevents the LH surge and ovulation from occurring. This is beneficial because premature ovulation can disrupt the carefully planned

treatment schedule and lead to the loss of the eggs before they can be retrieved.

The long protocol (i.e., Down regulation) requires the administration of GnRH agonists to begin one to two weeks *prior* to the start of ovarian stimulation to suppress hormone production from the brain, prevent premature ovulation, and allow for synchronized follicle development so they develop at a relatively even pace. Another protocol, the microdose flare, requires that GnRH agonists are administered at the start of the menstrual cycle along with gonadotropins as an extra "push" in follicle development. This protocol may be useful for women with diminished ovarian reserve and/or those who respond poorly to stimulation medications. In either protocol, GnRH agonist administration will cease prior to the egg retrieval.

Lupron can also be administered as a trigger shot instead of hCG to induce the final maturation of eggs before the retrieval. Lupron can reduce the risk of ovarian hyperstimulation syndrome (see below) compared to hCG. It may also be used in conjunction with hCG (a dual trigger) to prevent OHSS while ensuring effective egg maturation.

3. **GnRH antagonists** (Ganirelix, Cetrotide) are injectable medications that block the action of GnRH in the brain, which prevents the LH surge that triggers ovulation to occur. The goals of these medications are to extend the window of time for eggs to mature and prevent premature ovulation from occurring.

   GnRH antagonists are typically used during the later stages of ovarian stimulation in IVF (around the expected time of ovulation when the follicles are larger in diameter). Their administration helps to fine-tune the timing and maximize the chances of successful outcomes.

4. **Human Chorionic Gonadotropin** (hCG, Ovidrel, Pregnyl, Novarel, Profasi) is an intramuscular injectable medication that mimics the hormone LH and is used to trigger the final maturation of eggs and their release from the follicles (ovulation). This medication is typically prescribed roughly 34-36 hours prior to the egg retrieval. This gives the eggs optimal time to mature *without* causing ovulation to occur prior to the retrieval. Prior to administration, hCG must be mixed with a diluent to help maintain its stability and integrity.

5. **Progesterone** is a hormone that prepares the uterine lining for embryo implantation and supports early pregnancy. Progesterone can be administered as an intramuscular injection (often called PIO), vaginal suppository, skin patch, and/or gel during the IVF process.

Intramuscular injections are compounded in oil (sometimes peanut or sunflower, so be aware of peanut allergies).

For fresh embryo transfers, progesterone administration typically begins on the day of your egg retrieval. For frozen embryo transfers (FETs) progesterone is administered toward the middle of the menstrual cycle (around the time of ovulation) if the uterine lining is developing properly. FETs normally occur on the sixth day of progesterone administration (unless you are transferring day 3 embryos), though some variations exist.

Progesterone administration is continued until either:
- A negative pregnancy is confirmed
- The eighth to twelfth week of a confirmed pregnancy (timing can vary), which is when the placenta takes over progesterone production to sustain the pregnancy

6. **Estrogen** (Estrace) may also be prescribed to support the growth of the uterine lining in preparation for embryo transfer. It may be administered orally, transdermally, or vaginally.

Estrogen is typically administered at the start of an FET cycle (usually cycle day 3), and administration is continued along with progesterone. Both medications are typically discontinued at the same time (see above).

Minimal Stimulation

Minimal stimulation ("mini stim") IVF is an alternative approach to ovarian stimulation that uses lower doses of fertility medications compared to conventional protocols. The primary goal of minimal stimulation is to produce a smaller number of high-quality eggs while minimizing the risk of OHSS and reducing the cost and intensity of the treatment cycle.

Your fertility specialist may recommend minimal stimulation IVF for several reasons:

- Diminished ovarian reserve: Individuals with fewer eggs or reduced egg quality may benefit from minimal stimulation. Since their response to higher doses of medications is limited, using lower doses may still yield a small number of mature eggs while reducing the risk of complications.

- Lower risk of OHSS (see below): Mini stim protocols reduce the likelihood of overstimulating the ovaries.

- Personal preference: Some people prefer a more conservative approach with fewer injections, lower medication costs, and less physical strain.

It is important to note that minimal stimulation may result in fewer eggs retrieved than conventional protocols. However, the emphasis is on obtaining higher-quality eggs rather than maximizing quantity. Your fertility specialist will determine the most appropriate stimulation protocol based on your age, ovarian reserve, and treatment goals. It's crucial to have a detailed discussion with your fertility specialist to understand the potential benefits and limitations of minimal stimulation of this approach.

IVF Monitoring

Once you begin your IVF stimulation, you will return to your clinic for regular monitoring leading up to your egg retrieval. Monitoring typically includes an ultrasound scan of your ovaries and blood tests to evaluate you reproductive hormone levels.

While variations exist, most IVF clinics will perform baseline monitoring around day three of your menstrual cycle. Baseline monitoring normally consists of:

- An ultrasound to ensure that your ovaries and uterus are normal in appearance. An antral follicle count (AFC) can also be performed at this time, during which the number of small follicles (fluid-filled sacs that contain eggs) are counted to estimate how many eggs will mature and be available for IVF that cycle.

- Blood work to ensure that your reproductive hormone levels are within proper ranges.

If these results are normal, you will begin (or continue) administering medications according to your specialist's orders. Additional monitoring appointments are scheduled over the next approximately 8–12 days to ensure that your follicles (eggs) are developing and hormone levels are rising appropriately. Medication dosages can be adjusted as needed during this time based on these results.

Once some or all of the developing follicles reach a certain diameter (usually 15 mm or more) and your hormone levels are within specific ranges, you will be instructed to administer your trigger medication approximately thirty-four to thirty-six hours prior to your scheduled egg retrieval procedure. Your clinic will provide specific timing and instructions.

Medication Side Effects

Like any other medications, fertility medications can cause side effects, which specific side effects experienced may vary depending on the individual, medication type, and dosage. It's important to remember that these side effects are temporary but should be taken seriously. Common side effects include:

- **Injection site reactions**: injectable medications may cause pain, redness, swelling, or bruising at the injection site.
- **Ovarian Hyperstimulation Syndrome (OHSS)**: OHSS can occur as a result of ovarian stimulation, particularly when high doses of gonadotropins are used. It can cause enlarged ovaries, abdominal discomfort or bloating, nausea, vomiting, and in rare cases, fluid accumulation in the abdomen or chest. Severe cases of OHSS can cause shortness of breath and require medical attention.
- Hot flashes and mood swings
- Irritability
- Breast tenderness
- Headaches
- Nausea and vomiting
- Fatigue
- Abdominal discomfort, bloating, cramping, or pelvic pressure
- Dizziness

Birth Control and Fertility Treatment

It may seem counterintuitive, but birth control pills are commonly prescribed as part of fertility treatment protocols. Their use serves specific purposes that help optimize treatment outcomes. Here are a few reasons why birth control pills may be prescribed:

- **Ovarian suppression**: Birth control pills to temporarily suppress ovarian activity. This is particularly relevant in cases where your menstrual cycle needs to be regulated or synchronized with your treatment cycle. By taking birth control pills, the natural hormonal fluctuations of your menstrual cycle are suppressed, allowing for better control and timing of your following treatment steps.

- **Cycle scheduling**: Birth control pills provide a predictable and controlled menstrual cycle, enabling your fertility specialist to plan your treatment steps around a known starting point (e.g., withdrawal bleeding after stopping the pills). This allows your fertility specialist to optimize the timing of your medication administration, monitoring, and other procedures during your treatment cycle.
- **Follicle recruitment**: In some cases, a process called "flare protocol" or "estrogen priming" may be used. This involves briefly using birth control pills to suppress your ovarian activity, followed by a quick withdrawal to induce a rebound effect. The sudden drop in estrogen levels can stimulate the recruitment of a larger cohort of follicles, potentially increasing the chances of a successful egg retrieval and IVF cycle.
- **Cyst prevention**: Birth control pills can suppress your ovarian activity, which helps prevent the development of cysts on your ovaries that may interfere with your treatment.

It's important to note that all birth control pills are not created equal; some are made with different amounts of hormones in each pill. For an IVF cycle, it's common to use "monophasic" birth control pills that contain the same amount of hormone in each pill. This will help you maintain the same hormone level each day. The last row of pills are placebo pills, which contain no hormones. Your fertility specialist may instruct you to skip the placebo pills and continue with active pills only depending on your medical history and treatment plan. As with any medication, you will need to follow your fertility specialist's explicit instructions when administering birth control pills to optimize your chances of success.

It's encouraged that you take your pill at the same time each day. It might help to take the pill in the evening and with food to help reduce nausea. If you accidentally miss or skip a dose, reach out to your care team for guidance. Smoking should be avoided while taking birth control pills due to the increased risk of developing blood clots.

Although birth control pills are a very common medication used in IVF regimens, they may not be appropriate for everyone. Some people are unable to use it because they may have a certain blood clotting disorder or a low ovarian reserve. In this case, specialists may have patients use estrogen patches instead to help the ovaries prepare for stimulation.

Fertility Medication Considerations

Fertility medications most likely are a significant portion of your treatment costs. It helps to educate yourself and take the time to understand the storage recommendations, purpose, dosage, administration instructions, and possible side effects of each medication that you will be taking. It is also very important to follow the instructions provided by your fertility clinic regarding the administration, dosage, and timing of your medications. Here are some other tips to help you navigate the process:

- Set reminders or alarms on your phone so you don't miss any doses. Timing is critical for many fertility medications.
- Keep all of your supplies organized as soon as they arrive. Make sure refrigerated medications are put away before they get too warm.
- Maintain an adequate supply of medication on hand to avoid running out.
- Watch videos about how to administer each medication so you feel confident administering them.
- If you are uncomfortable administering medications, ask a support person or medical professional for help.
- Contact your clinic if you miss a dose or experience any concerning side effects. You care team can provide guidance and determine if any adjustments or interventions are necessary.

Elizabeth's Story

Deciding to do IVF (in vitro fertilization) was a BIG decision. In my eyes, this was a path that I did not want to go down. But, when you are left with not a lot of choices, the decision is practically made for you.

Once we signed our consents, we were ready to move forward with our IVF cycle. The first step was ordering our IVF medications. I was lucky because my insurance helped cover some, but not all, of the costs. As you may have heard, IVF is not cheap even with insurance. But we kept telling ourselves that it will eventually be worth it.

The pharmacy mailed me all of my medications in a cardboard box. When I opened the box, I almost cried. I had no idea what this stuff was and what it was being used for. I was so overwhelmed, especially since I had no medical background.

Thankfully, we scheduled a Zoom call with a nurse who explained everything and showed me exactly what I needed to do. I would definitely recommend doing this because I felt so much better afterward. It was also recorded so we could look back at it when we needed to.

PRO TIP: Order yourself an IVF medication storage bin! This REALLY helped me stay organized and on top of when to take and reorder my medications. You need to be really organized during IVF because if you run out of medications, it can impact your cycle.

Once we got our medications situated, we had to wait for my period to start my injections. This was very daunting to me because I am not a fan of needles. Did I mention that these had to be injected into my stomach? Not a fun time, but you have to do what you have to do.

The point of all these injections was to stimulate my ovaries to produce as many eggs as possible for the egg retrieval. It started with two injections each night and then increased to three as my cycle progressed. This whole process is time sensitive, and we would do injections at 8:00 p.m. every night. This meant that we had to be home by 7:45 p.m. to prepare the shots and get everything ready.

I felt like a nurse and chemist since I was mixing the medications and drawing them up into syringes. I was so nervous I was going to mess something up since this was not my area of expertise. The injections were definitely not fun, but they had to be done. I felt so bloated and uncomfortable. I was very hormonal and more moody than normal. The injections resulted in bruises all over my stomach, even though we alternated injection sites. But somehow we made it through this process and were able to move forward with not one, but two, IVF cycles. In the end, it was worth every shot.

One thing that really helped me through this process was having an amazing support system. My husband, family, and a select few friends were privy to what we were going through. This really helped me believe in myself and see the end of the finish line.

What I am trying to say is: you've got this. This community has the best members and people who are always willing to listen and give advice.

I hope that my story helps others realize what they are capable of doing and that they are a lot stronger mentally and physically than they might think.

Conclusions

Fertility treatment involves a wide range of medications, each tailored to your specific diagnosis, protocol, and medical history. Your fertility specialist will guide you through the most appropriate medication regimen to support your treatment goals. Understanding the purpose and timing of each medication empowers you to take an active role in your care and navigate the process with confidence.

Chapter 7
In Vitro Fertilization (IVF)

The information in this chapter was contributed by Jessica Manns, MS, embryologist and creator of ExplainingIVF

The Centers for Disease Control and Prevention (CDC) defines assisted reproductive technology (ART) as any fertility treatment or procedure in which eggs and/or embryos are handled outside of the body to help achieve pregnancy.[1] The most common form of ART is in vitro fertilization (IVF), which involves retrieving eggs (also called oocytes or ova) from the ovaries, fertilizing them with sperm in a laboratory, and transferring resulting embryos into the uterus of the intended parent (mother) or a gestational carrier (surrogate) in an attempt to initiate a pregnancy. Since the birth of the first IVF baby, Louise Joy Brown, in 1978, IVF has led to the birth of more than 12 million babies worldwide.

Though it sounds fairly straightforward, IVF is a complex, multistep process that can differ from person to person. In other words, some optional or alternative steps are not routinely performed unless they are necessary. Your fertility specialist will create a personalized treatment plan based on your diagnosis and medical history to optimize your chances of success. *Keep in mind that each clinic may have its own protocols and may perform the following steps differently than described in this chapter.*

An IVF cycle begins with the administration of medications and routine monitoring (see Chapter 6). The final portion of this phase involves the administration of a trigger medication, which causes the eggs to finish maturing in the ovaries and controls the timing of ovulation so it does not occur before the egg retrieval procedure, which is normally scheduled thirty-four to thirty-six hours after the trigger medication is administered. If ovulation occurs before the procedure, the eggs cannot be retrieved.

The Egg Retrieval Procedure

As its name suggests, the goal of an egg retrieval (also called an ovum pick up (OPU) or vaginal oocyte retrieval (VOR)) is to retrieve eggs from the ovaries. The retrieved eggs can then either be inseminated or frozen for future use. Recall from Chapter 3 that each egg resides in a fluid-filled sac called a follicle. While eggs are too small to be seen on an ultrasound scan, large follicles can be visualized and targeted during the procedure (Figure 7.1).

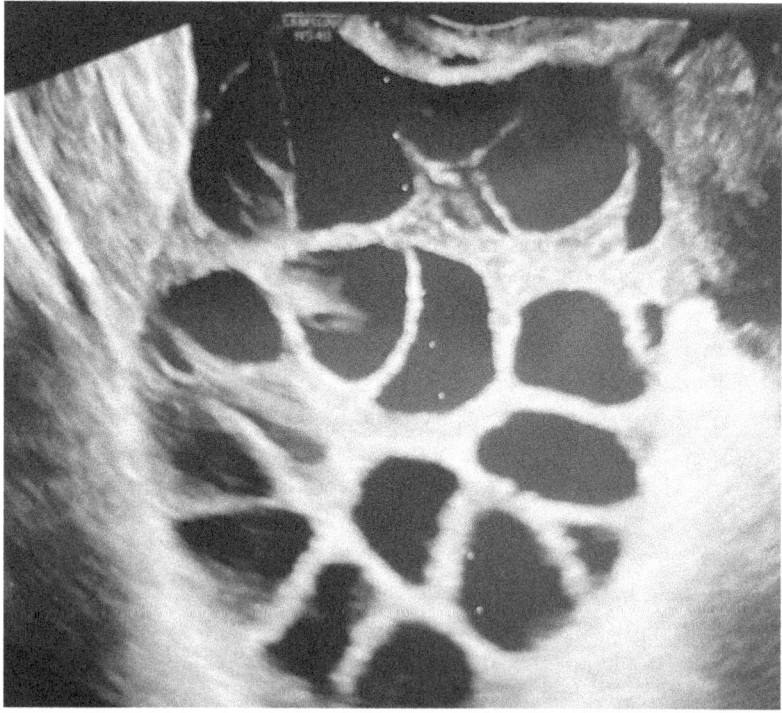

Figure 7.1 An ultrasound image of ovarian follicles.

Preparing for an Egg Retrieval

Your clinic should provide you with specific instructions to prepare for your egg retrieval, which may include:

- Do not eat or drink anything after midnight the night before your retrieval.
- Arrive thirty to sixty minutes prior to your scheduled start time (timing varies between clinics).
- Bring a support person to accompany you and drive you home after the retrieval if you will be under sedation (most egg retrievals are performed under sedation).
- Plan to take the rest of the day off to rest and recover.
- Talk with your fertility specialist about any medications that you will need to take before the retrieval.

When you arrive and check in for your egg retrieval, you will be directed to a private area to change into a clean gown. You (and your support person, if applicable) will have the opportunity to speak with a nurse and/or physician about your procedure and treatment plan, and you may need to sign additional consents. If you are receiving intravenous (IV) sedation, the IV will be placed at this time. You will then be escorted to the operating room (OR) with a staff member. Support people are not permitted in the OR during egg retrievals.

Once you are in the OR, your identity and treatment plan should be confirmed. A staff member will position you on the exam table while the fertility specialist thoroughly scrub his/her hands and arms. For this procedure, you will lie on your back with your feet in stirrups as if you are having a pelvic exam. Egg retrievals are usually performed under deep sedation, which helps you sleep or feel very relaxed. You'll be closely monitored by a medical professional throughout the procedure to ensure your safety and comfort.

During the Procedure

Egg retrievals are minimally invasive and are normally completed in about fifteen to thirty minutes, though timing may vary depending on the number of large follicles and the position of the ovaries. Egg retrievals are low-risk procedures, but antibiotics may be prescribed to mitigate the risk of acquiring an infection.

Once you are sedated, a speculum is inserted and the vaginal area is cleaned to minimize your risk of infection. A covered ultrasound probe is then inserted into your vagina to visualize the follicles in your ovaries, and the image is projected onto a screen in the OR. A needle that is attached to the ultrasound probe is then inserted through the wall of your vagina and into one of your ovaries. This needle is connected to a catheter (plastic tubing) and suction device, which generates gentle suction to aspirate (suck up) the fluid and eggs from the follicles (Figure 7.2).

Using the ultrasound as a guide, the physician will pierce each of your follicles and use the suction device to aspirate the contents of each enlarged follicle. As this occurs, the follicle typically collapses on the ultrasound screen. This is repeated for each enlarged follicle in both of your ovaries. The aspirated fluid travels through the catheter and is emptied into a sterile tube. Once a tube is filled, it is transferred to the IVF lab for inspection.

Once each large follicle has been aspirated, the needle, ultrasound probe, and speculum are removed. Some clinics allow you to recover in the OR, while

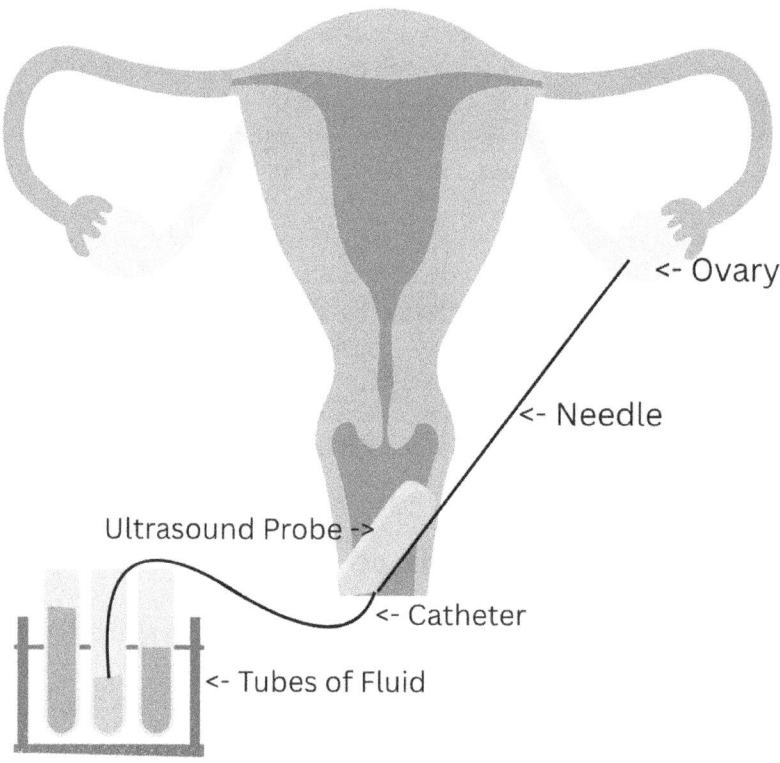

Figure 7.2 The egg retrieval procedure setup.

other clinics transfer you to a separate, private area to recover. The recovery process takes about forty-five minutes as your sedation wears off, and you are carefully monitored until you are ready to leave. Before you leave, you should be provided with your discharge instructions, restrictions, and next steps. Most clinics will follow up with you the next day to check on your recovery and discuss preliminary results.

The Egg Retrieval Process in the Lab

In the IVF lab, an embryologist empties the contents of each sterile tube into a sterile dish, and each dish is carefully examined under a microscope for eggs. Eggs normally appear as dark circles surrounded by fluffy cumulus cells (cells that nourish the egg in the follicle) (Figure 7.3). Eggs that are found are transferred to a clean holding dish, and the remaining fluid is discarded. This process is completed for each tube. Many labs also inspect each tube for retained eggs before discarding the tubes to ensure that none are missed.

Once all of the eggs have been isolated into a holding dish, the majority of the cumulus cells can be carefully trimmed from around each egg using a needle (Figure 7.4). This makes the eggs easier to count and handle.

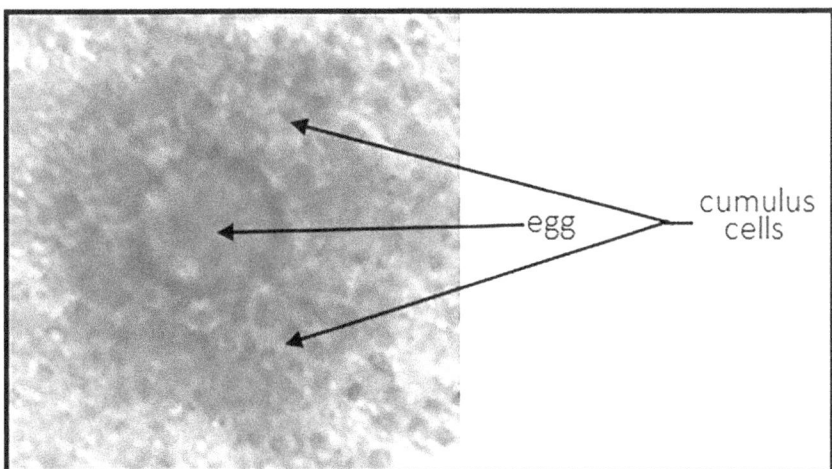

Figure 7.3 The cumulus oophorous complex (COC) consists of an egg (oocyte) surrounded by cumulus cells. The innermost layer of cumulus cells is called the corona radiata.

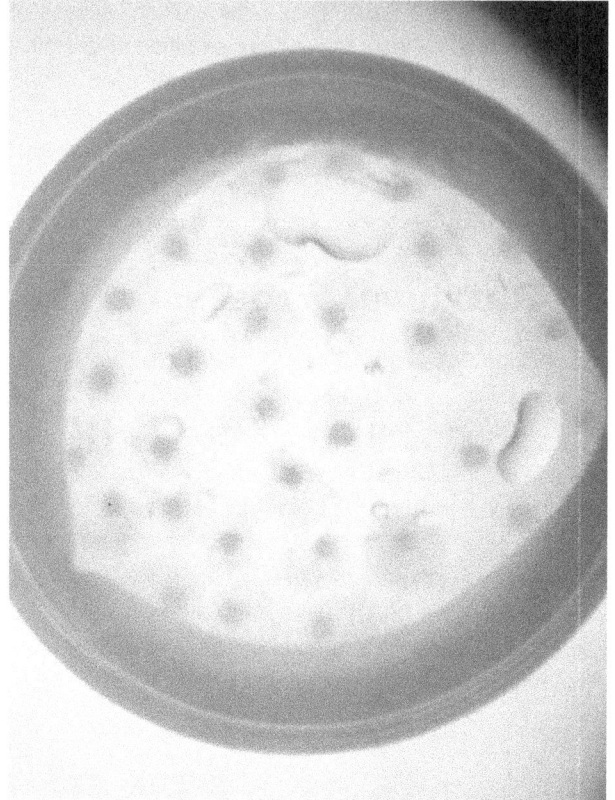

Figure 7.4 Eggs (oocytes) after the removal of excess cumulus cells.

From this point, two possible events can occur:

1. The eggs are placed into a medium (fluid) that contains the enzyme hyaluronidase. The cumulus cells surrounding eggs are bound together by a substance called hyaluronic acid. Hyaluronidase breaks down hyaluronic acid, which loosens the bonds between the cumulus cells. The eggs are carefully pipeted up and down using specialized pipettes with decreasing diameters to gently remove the remaining cumulus cells from around them. Eggs are only exposed to hyaluronidase for a short period of time before they are transferred to a different medium and ultimately placed into a culture dish (a labeled dish that contains specialized culture medium that supports egg/sperm/embryo development) in an incubator. This process, known as egg stripping or denudation, is performed if the eggs are being frozen (vitrified) or undergoing intracytoplasmic sperm injection (ICSI), but not conventional insemination.

2. The eggs are placed into a culture dish inside an incubator. The temperature and gas concentrations in incubators are programmed to create an environment that mimics the female reproductive tract to support optimal development. This would occur if the eggs are:

   a. Being stripped at a later time (some clinics wait to strip eggs) prior to ICSI or egg freezing.

   b. Undergoing conventional insemination (IVF) and do not require stripping.

Eggs are frozen or inseminated a few hours after they are retrieved.

Frozen eggs are thawed (warmed) a few hours prior to insemination (timing varies between labs). Thawed eggs must undergo ICSI since their cumulus cells are removed before they are frozen and their shells (zona pellucidae) harden during the freezing process. See below for more information about thawing.

Egg Maturity

After the eggs are stripped for freezing or ICSI, they are separated based on their (nuclear) maturity.

As discussed in Chapter 3, eggs are formed inside follicles in the ovaries during early fetal development. These immature eggs begin the process of meiosis, a specialized type of cell division that halves the number of chromosomes (genetic material) in the egg, but the process is halted early on. At the beginning of each menstrual cycle, a group of eggs resumes meiosis. However, only one (occassionally two or more) egg in the group reaches full maturity while the others degenerate. This is the egg that is ovulated during that menstrual cycle. Ovarian stimulation medications cause multiple eggs to mature simultaneously instead of just one.

Eggs actually undergo two meiotic (cell) divisions. The first division (meiosis 1) begins during fetal development but is not completed until just before ovulation or an egg retrieval. We will discuss the second meiotic division below. When the egg divides, a small, nonfunctional cell called a polar body forms next to the egg. Thus, embryologists know that an egg has completed its first meiotic division if there is a polar body present (Figure 7.5). Only eggs that have completed meiosis 1 are able to be fertilized. They are considered mature and are often referred to as M2 oocytes.

On average, 70–80 percent of retrieved eggs are mature even with the administration of ovarian stimulation medications, though this number can vary based on a number of factors.

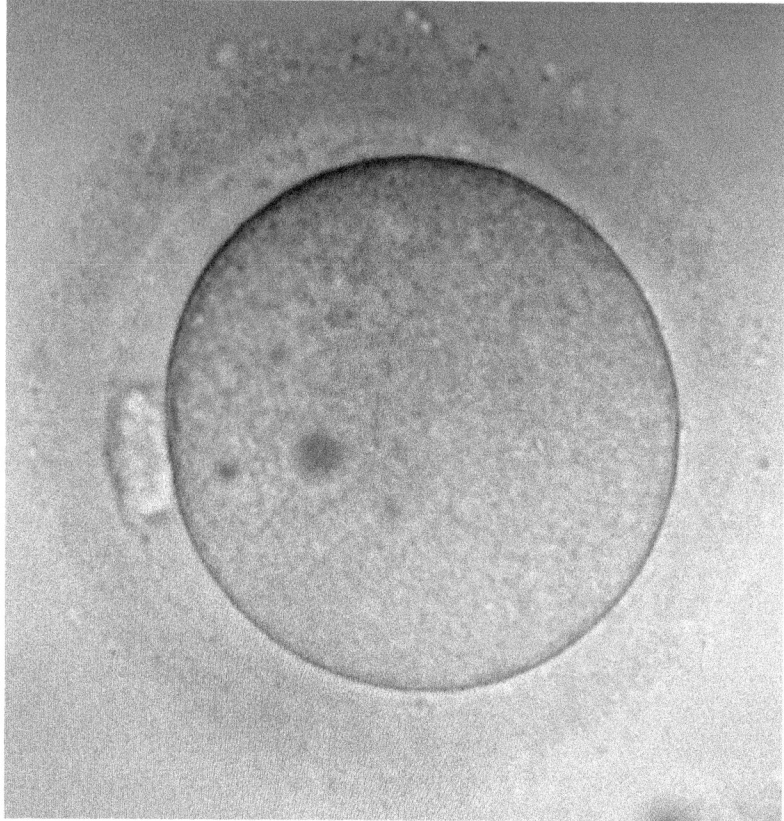

Figure 7.5 A mature egg (M2).

In addition to mature eggs, it's possible to retrieve:

- **M1 oocytes**: immature eggs that have not completed their first meiotic division and do not contain a polar body. They may complete meiosis 1 within a few hours.
- **Germinal vesicles (GVs)**: very immature eggs with a visible nucleus. They will not complete meiosis 1 for a long period of time (or ever).
- **Degenerate (atretic or nonviable) eggs**
- **Empty or fractured zonas**: only a shell (zona pellucida) is present without an egg inside
- **Abnormal eggs** (e.g., an egg composed of two cells)
- **Diploid eggs**: large eggs with an extra set of chromosomes due to abnormal cell division

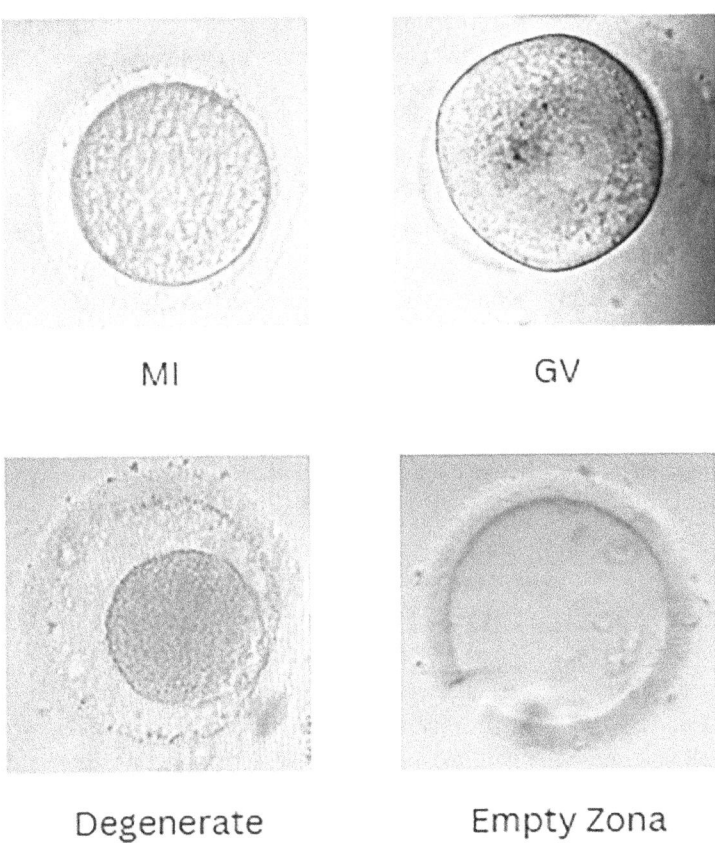

Figure 7.6 An immature egg (MI), germinal vesicle (GV), degenerate egg, and empty zona pellucida (shell).

Typically, GVs, degenerate eggs, fractured or empty zonas, and diploid eggs are discarded. Some clinics may also discard abnormal eggs depending on the type and severity of the abnormality. MI oocytes are sometimes given a few hours to mature to M2s. If they do, they can be frozen or inseminated (depending on your clinic's policy).

In Vitro Maturation

In vitro maturation (IVM) is the process of retrieving immature eggs from their follicles in the ovaries (or entire segments of the ovaries, which should contain immature eggs) and allowing them to mature in the lab for varying lengths of time. If these eggs do mature, they can be frozen or inseminated via ICSI.

Since IVM requires little to no ovarian stimulation, it is typically reserved for those with a high risk of developing ovarian hyperstimulation syndrome (OHSS) or certain health conditions such as cancers that could be worsened by excessive hormone administration.

Compared to traditional IVF, IVM is cost-effective and can help limit the number of medications that must be administered during IVF stimulation. However, though eggs that mature through IVM have the ability to result in healthy live births, they yield lower live birth rates compared to oocytes that are mature at the time of retrieval. This may be due to incomplete cytoplasmic maturation, which involves metabolic and structural changes within the egg that prepare it for fertilization and development. This is different than nuclear maturation and cannot be visualized.

Some labs routinely perform IVM, while others do not. While IVM currently isn't as effective as traditional IVF, ongoing advancements in IVM techniques are promising.[2]

Many Immature Eggs Retrieved

Egg maturation is a complex process involving precise gene expression, cytoplasmic maturation, and other events that must occur at very specific times. Even with the administration of ovarian stimulation medications, there are some situations in which most (or all) of the eggs that are retrieved are immature.

Some eggs do not mature due to[3]:

- An inadequate response to the IVF stimulation medications
- Incorrect dosage or timing of the trigger medication
- A stimulation cycle that was too short (the eggs needed more time to mature)
- The specific stimulation protocol used (i.e., the types and dosages of medications that were administered)
- Polycystic ovary syndrome (PCOS)
- Diminished ovarian reserve (DOR)
- Primary ovarian insufficiency (POI) and/or high FSH levels
- Advanced maternal age, though immature eggs can be retrieved at any age
- Genetic abnormalities in the eggs
- Thyroid dysfunction
- Insulin resistance

- Poor ovarian blood flow
- Endometriosis
- Chronic stress

In some situations, changes can be made to future IVF cycles to yield more mature eggs. For example, different medication types and/or dosages may be administered, or the stimulation can be pushed for an additional day to allow more time for the eggs to mature. Unfortunately, these alterations cannot always guarantee a different outcome in a subsequent cycle.

Some labs give immature eggs a few hours to mature after they have been retrieved. If they mature in this time, they are able to be frozen or inseminated via ICSI. Some labs also offer day 1 ICSI, in which immature eggs are given a day to mature. If they mature, they can be inseminated the day after the egg retrieval. Embryos from day 1 ICSI have lower success rates compared to embryos from day 0 ICSI, but healthy live births have been reported following day 1 ICSI.

Empty Follicles

During IVF monitoring, the number of large follicles and blood hormone levels are used to predict the number of eggs that will be retrieved. However, sometimes fewer eggs are collected than expected. In these situations, follicles grow in size but no eggs are retrieved from them. Thus, they are referred to as empty follicles.

It's estimated that up to 20 percent of enlarged follicles will not contain an egg, but empty follicles are most commonly observed in individuals with PCOS and diminished ovarian reserve (DOR). In rare cases, no eggs are retrieved even if follicles are present. This is known as empty follicle syndrome (EFS).

Possible causes of empty follicles include[4]:

- Ovulation occurred too early and the eggs were expelled from their follicles
- The trigger medication was administered improperly or at the wrong time
- The eggs adhered to the wall of their follicles and could not be retrieved (eggs should detach from the walls of their follicles during their final stages of maturation)
- Poor ovarian response to the medications or abnormal response to hCG
- The eggs degenerated before they could be retrieved
- Structural abnormalities within the ovary, follicle, and/or egg
- Technical issues with the egg retrieval equipment (rare)

Depending on the cause, adjustments may be made in future IVF cycles (e.g., modifying medication protocols or timing) to reduce the likelihood of empty follicles. If this applies to you, talk with your fertility specialist about your options.

Egg Freezing (Oocyte Cryopreservation) and Thawing

There is a steady increase in the number of people who are freezing their eggs. The most common technique for egg freezing is called vitrification, which replaced a less efficient method known as slow freezing. An egg freezing cycle begins the same way as an IVF cycle: ovarian stimulation medications are administered and eggs are retrieved and graded based on their maturity. Egg freezing typically occurs on the same day as an egg retrieval, though some clinics may freeze eggs that need more time to mature the following day, as well. Some clinics only freeze mature eggs, while a few will also freeze immature eggs (this is typically reserved for patients who freeze their eggs for medical reasons, such as cancer treatment).

Egg freezing involves moving eggs through a series of media that remove water from the eggs and coat them with a cryoprotectant agent (see "Embryo Freezing" section below for more information). This agent prevents ice crystals from forming, which could damage the egg. The eggs are then placed on labeled, specialized devices and stored in liquid nitrogen for future use.

There are many reasons why people freeze their eggs, including:

- Elective fertility preservation
- Egg donation
- Medical treatments (e.g., chemotherapy, radiation therapy, or certain gender-affirming surgeries)
- Medical conditions (e.g., DOR or POI)
- A family history of primary ovarian insufficiency (POI)
- Lack of sperm at the time of insemination
- High egg yield with a desire to limit the number of embryo created

Eggs can remain frozen indefinitely. The thawing process involves removing the eggs from liquid nitrogen and moving them through media that remove the cryoprotectant agent and safely reintroduce water to the eggs.

In general, roughly 90–95 percent of eggs frozen via vitrification survive the freezing and thawing processes (the survival rate is lower for slow frozen eggs), though each clinic may have its own rate. Keep in mind that eggs only consist of one cell and are more fragile than embryos, which have higher survival rates. The number of eggs you should freeze depends on your age, medical history, and family-building goals.

After the eggs are thawed, they are inseminated via ICSI and progress through an IVF cycle in the same manner as fresh (unfrozen) eggs. Fertilization and clinical pregnancy rates are similar between fresh and frozen eggs.

Sperm Information

Spermatozoa (sperm) are the male gametes, or sex cells, that fertilize eggs to create embryos. Recall from Chapter 2 that sperm production should occur in the testes from the onset of puberty and continue throughout a male's life.

Sperm Collection

Sperm are most commonly collected through ejaculation. For clinical purposes, a male will ejaculate into a sterile specimen cup either at home or a fertility clinic. The sample should be properly verified by a staff member at the clinic before it is released from the male's custody. The semen sample is analyzed and, if applicable, processed for insemination or freezing (cryopreservation).

In cases where sperm are produced but not present in the ejaculate, surgical retrieval may be necessary. Procedures include:

- **Percutaneous epididymal sperm aspiration (PESA)**: a small needle is inserted into the epididymis to aspirate (suck up) sperm present inside of it.
- **Microsurgical epididymal sperm aspiration (MESA):** a small incision is made in the scrotum, and a microscope is used to visualize portions of the epididymis where sperm are most likely present. A small incision is made in this area, and the fluid (and hopefully sperm) is aspirated from it.
- **Testicular sperm aspiration (TESA)**: a small needle is inserted into the seminiferous sample is in the testes to aspirate sperm from the tubules.
- **Testicular sperm extraction (TESE)**: a small sample of the seminiferous tubules (and hopefully sperm) are surgically removed from the testes. The tubules are then processed in the lab to identify and extract viable sperm.

- **Microdissection-TESE (micro-TESE)**: an incision is made in one or both testicles, and a trained physician uses a microscope to find swollen seminiferous tubules that are most likely to contain sperm. These tubules are surgically removed and processed in the lab to identify and extract viable sperm.

The procedure type depends on the reason why sperm is not present in the ejaculate. Keep in mind that each of these techniques may require multiple attempts to retrieve enough sperm for insemination, and, in some cases, no sperm will be retrieved.

Sperm Preparation

Ejaculated semen normally contains millions of sperm and seminal fluid, which nourishes suspended in protects the sperm. A semen sample may contain sperm that:

- Are normal or abnormal in appearance
- Are motile or nonmotile
- Have intact or fragmented DNA

When sperm enter the female reproductive tract, motile sperm are naturally separated from nonmotile or nonviable sperm and other contents of the semen on their way to the egg.

For IUIs or IVF, healthy sperm must be mechanically isolated from immotile or nonviable sperm and other contents of the semen outside of the body. This process, known as sperm preparation, washing, or processing, isolates high-quality sperm for use in fertility treatment. There are three common sperm preparation methods:

- **Density gradient centrifugation (DGC).** A liquefied semen sample is placed into a sterile tube on top of fluids with different densities. This mixture is centrifuged (spun really fast), causing motile sperm (with slightly higher densities) to swim through the media to the bottom of the tube while the remaining seminal constituents are trapped at the top. The result should be a pellet of motile sperm at the bottom of the tube (Figure 7.7). The excess fluid (supernatant) is removed from above the pellet, and the pellet is typically placed into a new sterile tube with new fluid and centrifuged again. Regardless, the final sperm sample is ultimately placed into a labeled tube for fertility treatment.

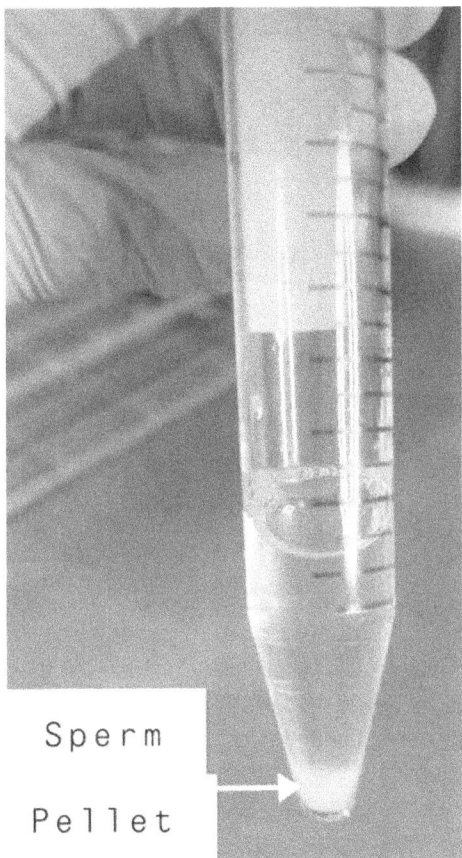

Figure 7.7 A sperm pellet following centrifugation of the semen sample.

- **Swim-up method.** A liquefied semen sample is placed into the bottom of an angled sterile tube and overlaid with a specialized fluid for thirty or more minutes (timing varies) at approximately 37°C (Figure 7.8). During this time, motile sperm swim to the top of the fluid while the nonmotile sperm and other seminal constituents remain at the bottom of the tube. The upper layer of the fluid, which should contain only motile sperm, is then removed and placed into a sterile labeled tube for fertility treatment. Some clinics may centrifuge the initial and/or final samples, as well.
- **Sperm Separation Devices (ZyMōt™, LensHooke® CA0, SwimCount® Harvester).** These commercially available devices are increasing in popularity among IVF clinics. To operate these devices, semen is loaded into a lower chamber and specialized fluid is loaded into an upper collection chamber of the device. The device is placed in a

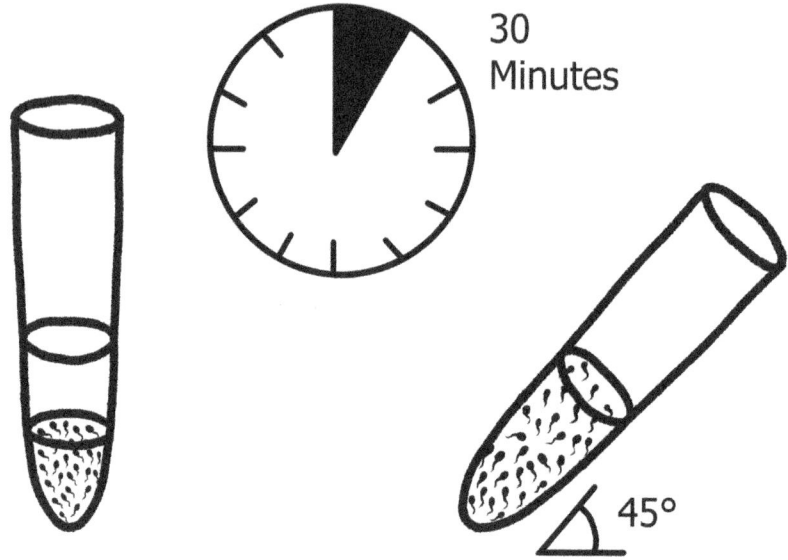

Figure 7.8 The swim-up method.

warm environment for thirty minutes, during which the motile sperm swim upward through barriers (these vary between devices) into the upper chamber. Afterward, a sample that should contain fluid and motile sperm is collected from the upper chamber. Many labs analyze the sperm in this sample before placing the sample into a sterile, labeled tube for fertility treatment.

Multiple studies have found that, compared to other methods of sperm preparation, sperm separation devices can lead to lower levels of sperm DNA fragmentation,[5] which in turn may increase euploidy, implantation, and live birth rates, though more studies are needed.

Keep in mind that each clinic may have its own policies regarding sperm preparation. Some clinics may offer multiple options, while others may only routinely perform one of the above methods.

Freezing Sperm

It's possible and fairly easy to freeze (cryopreserve) sperm for future use. This procedure involves placing a portion of a sperm sample into a labeled plastic cryovial along with a specialized cryoprotectant solution that protects the sperm during freezing. Multiple vials can be frozen at once and are typically secured to a metal cane (Figure 7.9). Various freezing protocols exist, but the vials are ultimately plunged into liquid nitrogen, which remains around −196°C. All cellular activity is halted while the sperm remain in liquid nitrogen, so they can be frozen

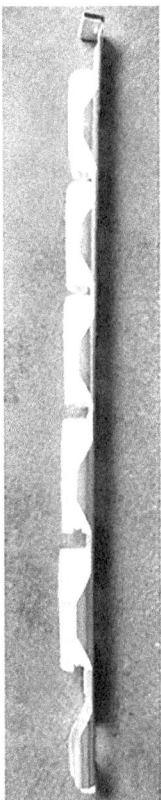

Figure 7.9 Sperm cryovials in a metal cane.

indefinitely. Some clinics wash sperm before it is frozen, while other clinics wait to wash the sperm until after it is thawed—both approaches are valid and depend on clinic policy and intended use.

There are many reasons why sperm may be frozen for future use, including:

- Upcoming medical treatments (e.g., chemotherapy, radiation, or gender-affirming surgery) that can impair sperm production and quality
- Inability to produce a fresh semen sample on the day of insemination
- Sperm donation (sperm is frozen and donated to another individual or couple)
- A desire to have backup sperm available for fertility treatment
- Personal reasons, such as advanced age or anxiety about producing a sample at a specific time

In rare cases, sperm can be collected 1 to 3 days after death through a procedure known as posthumous sperm retrieval (PSR). This requires legal documentation and is typically performed with the consent of the deceased's family or partner. PSR is a highly specialized process and may not be available at all clinics.[6]

Insemination and Fertilization

Insemination is the process of introducing sperm to an egg for fertilization purposes (see Chapter 3). In an IVF lab, two primary types of insemination are used:

1. **Conventional insemination (IVF):** Though it occurs inside culture medium (fluid) in a dish within an incubator, IVF is similar to *in vivo* conception in the fallopian tube: multiple sperm attempt to penetrate the corona radiata (layer of cumulus cells surrounding the egg) and egg's shell (zona pellucida). One sperm then fuses with the egg's inner plasma membrane to initiate oocyte activation and hopefully achieve fertilization. IVF requires many sperm to facilitate fertilization, so it is not recommended in cases of low sperm count, motility, or abnormal morphology.

    Keep in mind that eggs are not cleaned and graded based on their maturity prior to IVF. This means that *all* of the retrieved eggs are placed into a culture medium with sperm overnight. Some retrieved eggs may not be mature, and only mature eggs can be fertilized. Thus, more eggs may enter the process, but fertilization rates may be lower than they are for ICSI (see below) since some of the eggs may not be mature at the time of insemination. The average fertilization rate with IVF is roughly 50 percent.

    A note about intravaginal culture (IVC): Intravaginal culture is a fertility treatment that uses a woman's vagina as a natural incubator for fertilization and early embryo development. It involves retrieving eggs and combining them (uncleaned and ungraded) with sperm in a small plastic capsule device (a common example is the INVOcell® device). Alternatively, a few clinics may clean and perform ICSI on the eggs before they are inserted into the device. This device is then inserted into the upper vagina for 3–5 days. After this time, the device is removed and the contents are inspected to see if any of the eggs fertilized and developed into embryos. These embryos can be transferred, frozen, or given a few days to develop in the lab. One study that accumulated data across four IVF clinics found an average live birth rate of 40–61 percent per transfer using INVOcell®.[7] IVC can alleviate some of the costs associated with IVF, but you and your fertility specialist should discuss whether IVC is an efficient option for you.

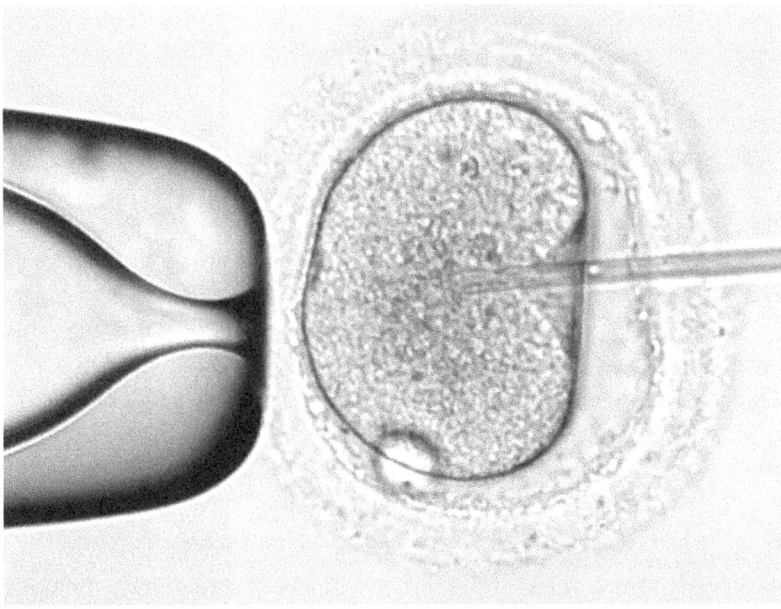

Figure 7.10 The injection of a sperm into a mature egg (oocyte) during intracytoplasmic sperm injection (ICSI).

2. **Intracytoplasmic sperm injection (ICSI)** involves injecting a single sperm into a mature egg (Figure 7.10). ICSI bypasses a sperm's need to swim to an egg, penetrate the corona radiata and zona pellucida, and fuse with the egg's plasma membrane. Thus, only one sperm is required to inseminate each egg, so ICSI is optimal in cases of low sperm count, motility, and/or morphology. Only mature eggs undergo ICSI since immature eggs cannot be fertilized.

   Embryologists inseminate eggs with sperm that are normal in appearance and motility for optimal success rates. Once a sperm is selected, its tail is gently kinked with the tip of a needle to immobilize it and disrupt its plasma membrane (in a good way) so that it can release substances that initiate oocyte activation once it enters the egg. Sperm are loaded into a specialized ICSI needle via controlled suction.

Once a sperm is loaded into the needle, an egg is held in place with gentle suction from a specialized holding pipette. The egg is maneuvered so the polar body is in the twelve or six o' clock position (though some labs prefer alternate placements), which minimizes the risk of damaging a structure in the egg called the meiotic spindle. Using reverse suction, the sperm is moved to the end of the ICSI needle. The needle is then injected through the zona pellucida until it reaches the plasma membrane. Suction is reapplied to the ICSI needle to break the plasma membrane. This ensures that the sperm is deposited inside the egg's ooplasm (the jelly-like substance within an egg that is often referred to as cytoplasm). Once the plasma membrane is broken, reverse suction is applied to deposit the sperm into the ooplasm, and then the ICSI needle is carefully removed.

ICSI has shown higher fertilization rates than IVF in cases of male factor infertility (e.g., a low sperm count or motility), unexplained infertility, or a history of poor or absent fertilization with conventional IVF. ICSI is also required for eggs that have been frozen[8]. Overall, fertilization rates with ICSI range from 50-80%, though this can vary between clinics and depends on many factors such as egg and sperm quality. ICSI also decreases the risk of cycle cancellation due to total fertilization failure (a situation in which no eggs fertilize). The downfalls of ICSI are that:

- It is more expensive and time consuming than conventional IVF.
- There is a small (<5 %) risk of damaging the egg during injection.
- Some studies suggest slightly increased risks of congenital anomalies (birth defects) such as urogenital or heart defects when ICSI is performed, though it's unclear if these are a direct result of ICSI or other factors such as embryo culture or the underlying cause of infertility.[9,10]
- ICSI may increase the risk of embryo splitting (twins, triplets, etc. resulting from one embryo).

Unlike most cells in our bodies that contain two sets of DNA, sperm and egg cells each carry one set. When insemination occurs, the sperm fuses with the egg's plasma membrane and deposits its single set of DNA into the egg. This triggers a series of events known as oocyte activation to occur, which includes:

- Calcium oscillations (calcium is repeatedly released from a structure in the egg known as the endoplasmic reticulum). This initiates a signaling cascade, activating various enzymes and cellular pathways within the egg.
- Release of enzymes that harden the egg's shell (zona pellucida), which blocks additional sperm from entering the egg (this is called the block to polyspermy).
- Completion of the egg's second meiotic cell division (the final stage of maturation), which results in the formation of a second polar body.
- Formation of the sperm and egg's pronuclei, which each consist of one set of DNA.

Eventually, the membranes of the sperm and egg's pronuclei fuse together to create a single nucleus. Inside of this nucleus are two sets of DNA (one from the sperm and one from the egg), so the embryo now has a full set of DNA.

Artificial Oocyte Activation (AOA)

Recall from above that calcium oscillations are an important initial step in oocyte activation and fertilization. Some clinics place inseminated eggs into a fluid containing calcium ionophores for approximately ten to fifteen minutes (timing may vary) following ICSI. This fluid allows increased levels of calcium to enter the egg to trigger oocyte activation. The inseminated eggs are then placed back into a culture medium overnight in an incubator. Studies have shown promising results with AOA when there is a history of poor or absent fertilization following ICSI.[11,12]

Physiological Intracytoplasmic Sperm Injection (PICSI)

PICSI is essentially the same process as ICSI, but it involves the additional step of exposing sperm to hyaluronic acid. The theory is that only mature sperm possess receptors that bind to hyaluronic acid, and mature sperm are less likely to have DNA fragmentation. Thus, only sperm that bind to the hyaluronic acid are selected for ICSI. Studies show conflicting results, with most finding no significant difference in live birth rates between PICSI and ICSI. In general, PICSI is not routinely used in IVF clinics and is typically reserved for situations with high levels of sperm DNA fragmentation and/or a history of poor fertilization with ICSI.[13]

Fertilization

Fertilization is a multistep biological process that results in the fusion of a sperm and egg's DNA (genetic material) to produce a single-cell embryo (zygote) with two sets of DNA. Regardless of whether conventional IVF or ICSI was performed, an embryologist will observe the inseminated eggs roughly sixteen to twenty hours after insemination (timing varies between labs) for signs of fertilization. Normal fertilization is confirmed by the presence of:

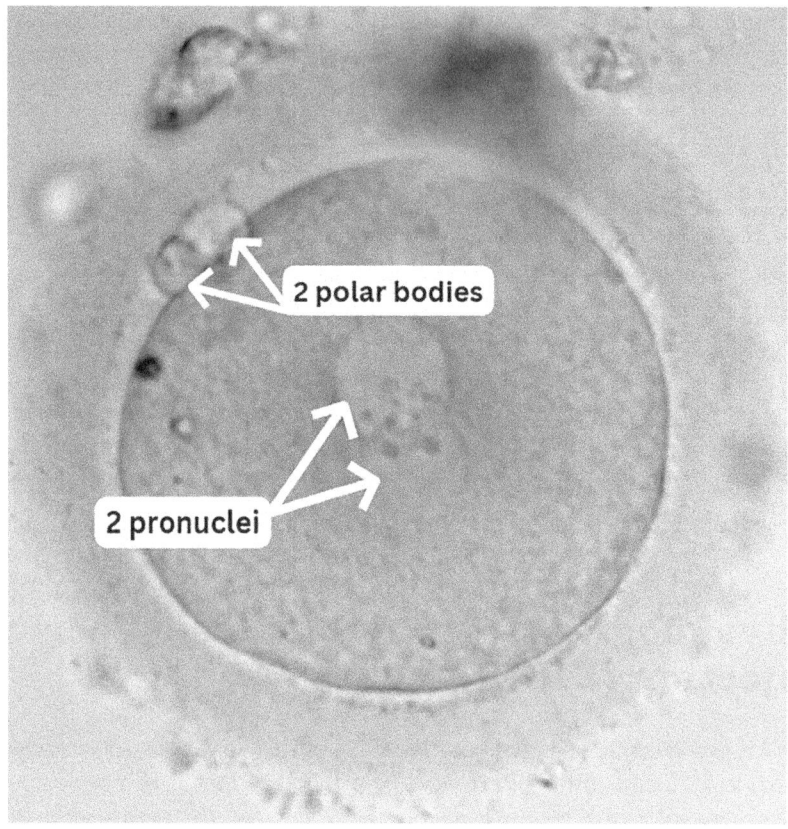

Figure 7.11 A fertilized egg contains two pronuclei and two polar bodies.

- **Two pronuclei** within the egg's ooplasm. One contains the set of DNA from the egg and the other contains the set of DNA from the sperm. The pronuclei eventually fuse together to create one nucleus, which will contain these two sets of DNA (this is called the embryo's genome). This becomes the genetic blueprint for the embryo, and every cell in the embryo *should* contain identical sets of DNA.
- **Two polar bodies** inside the shell (zona pellucida). This indicates that the egg has completed its second meiotic division, which cannot be completed unless fertilization occurs.

Some inseminated eggs may not show normal signs of fertilization. Other types of eggs that may be observed are:

- 0PN (no pronuclei are present)
- 1PN (one pronucleus, or one set of DNA, is present)

- 3PN (three pronuclei, or an extra set of DNA, are present)
- Degenerate (Atreticor nonviable)
- Abnormal (e.g., a two-cell embryo)

There are many reasons why eggs may not properly fertilize, including:

- With conventional insemination, it's possible that:
  - A sperm does not reach an egg and/or deposit its genetic material into the egg.
  - Some or all of the eggs are not mature (i.e., they are immature, degenerate, or abnormal). Recall that eggs are not graded based on their maturity prior to conventional IVF, and only mature eggs can be fertilized.
- Even if a sperm enters an egg, it may not deposit its DNA into the egg and/or the essential steps of oocyte activation still may not occur properly for multiple reasons. For example, the sperm's head may not decondense to release its DNA into the egg.
- Sperm and/or egg quality issues can cause fertilization to occur abnormally. This can be the case even if the egg or sperm appear normal. For example, impaired mitochondrial function (mitochondria provide the egg and sperm with energy) in the egg or sperm can interfere with normal fertilization.
- Polyspermy (multiple sperm may enter an egg and deposit their DNA into the egg). This causes the embryo to have an extra set of chromosomes.
- The sperm and/or egg have genetic abnormalities that cause errors in pronuclear formation and fertilization.
- Atresia (the egg does not survive the insemination process). This occurs in less than 5 percent of cases and typically occurs in eggs that are post-mature (too mature) or abnormally fragile.
- The egg activates but no sperm DNA is present.

Unfortunately, many of these abnormalities cannot be detected prior to insemination, making fertilization outcomes unpredictable. Some labs will allow eggs to develop even if they do not show proper signs of fertilization, while other labs will not.

Total fertilization failure occurs when no eggs that are inseminated show normal signs of fertilization. This occurs in 2–3 percent of ICSI cycles and 5–10 percent of conventional IVF cycles.[14]

Rescue ICSI

Some clinics may perform rescue ICSI, during which ICSI is performed on unfertilized eggs approximately eighteen to twenty-four hours following conventional IVF. Fertilization can occur following rescue ICSI and these embryos can result in healthy live births. However, it is recommended that these embryos are transferred via a frozen embryo transfer. Embryos created via rescue ICSI have average live birth rates (following frozen embryo transfers) of 46.7–47.53 percent, though outcomes may vary depending on individual factors and clinic protocols[15,16].

Embryo Development

Following fertilization, zygotes (fertilized eggs) are placed into droplets of culture fluid in a sterile dish. This dish is then placed into an incubator, which provides an environment that mimics the female reproductive tract. Over the course of 5–7 days (depending on your clinic's protocol), these embryos should develop from one to over 100 cells. This development occurs through a process known as mitosis, or cell division.

To review, the fertilized egg (zygote) consists of one cell with a set of DNA from both the sperm and egg. Over the course of roughly thirty hours, the zygote should divide into two cells (called blastomeres). During this process, the DNA inside of the zygote is replicated, and the new cell that is created receives one copy of that DNA, while the original cell retains one copy. The result is two cells that have identical DNA. These two cells then also undergo mitosis to result in four cells, and so on, all with the same DNA. Cells do not always divide at exactly the same pace, so it's possible to observe an uneven number of cells during the early stages of cell division.

Though each embryo develops at its own pace, there is a general timeline that embryos tend to follow:

Hours/Days After Insemination	Normal Developmental Stage	Description	Image
At fertilization	1 cell	A fertilized egg (zygote), see image above	
~30 hours	2 cells	The zygote undergoes one cell division, and the embryo enters the cleavage (cellular) stage of development.	
2 days	3-6 cells	The cleavage-stage embryo continues to undergo cell division, resulting in more cells (blastomeres) that continuously become smaller in size.	
3 days	6-12+ cells	The cleavage-stage embryo continues to undergo cell division, resulting in more cells (blastomeres) that continuously become smaller in size.	
	Early morula (EM)	The blastomeres begin to compact to form a structure known as an early morula.	

(Continued)

Hours/ Days After Insemination	Normal Developmental Stage	Description	Image
4 days	Morula (M)	The early morula becomes more compact.	
	Early blastocyst (EB)	A small cavity (blastocoel) forms inside the morula, which takes up <50% of the embryo's volume. The embryo enters the blastocyst stage of development.	
5 days	Blastocyst (B or BL)	The blastocoel expands and fills >50% of the embryo's volume. 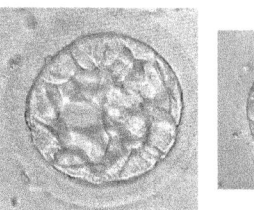	
	Full blastocyst (FB)	The blastocoel continues to expand and fill 100% of the embryo's volume. The embryo has not grown in diameter at this point. A clear inner cell mass and trophectoderm (see below) are now present in the embryo.	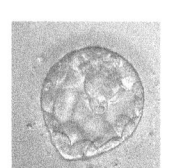

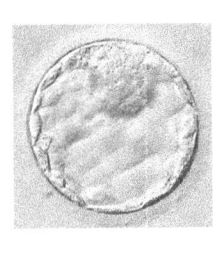

Expanded blastocyst
(XB or ExB)

The shell (zona pellucida) surrounding the embryo thins as the embryo expands in diameter. The embryo should consist of over 100 cells at this point and have a clear inner cell mass and trophectoderm.

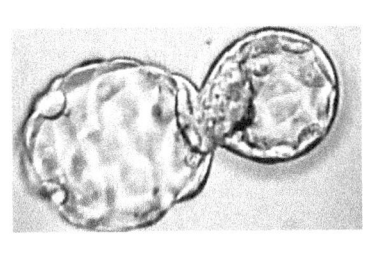

Hatching blastocyst (HgB)

A small hole forms in the zona pellucida, and the embryo begins to emerge from the hole.

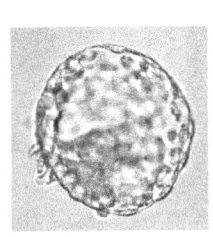

Hatched blastocyst
(HB or HdB)

The entire embryo has fully emerged from the zona pellucida, which is required for implantation.

6/7 days

Embryos that do not follow this exact timeline can still result in healthy live births. However, multiple studies have found that the slower the embryo's rate of development, the lower its overall chance of success. More specifically, embryos that are transferred, biopsied, and/or frozen 7 days after insemination ("day 7 embryos") yield lower implantation, pregnancy, and live birth rates compared to day 6 embryos, which in turn yield slightly lower overall success rates compared to day 5 embryos.[17,18,19] However, some studies have found no significant differences when a high-quality day 5 or 6 embryo is transferred.[20] Frozen embryo transfers are recommended when there is a delay in embryo development.

Developmental Arrest

On average, 30–50 percent of fertilized eggs will develop enough to be transferred, biopsied, and/or frozen (vitrified). Embryos that show no signs of development over at least twenty-four hours are considered arrested (not progressing). Embryo arrest is most common during the cleavage (cellular) stages of development and is believed to be a defense mechanism that prevents embryos with abnormalities from developing. However, there are many reasons why embryos arrest, including.[21,22]

- **Absent or abnormal genomic activation.** When eggs develop, they should contain genetic materials (particularly RNA) that drive early embryo development if the egg becomes fertilized. Even though an egg receives genetic material (DNA) from the sperm during fertilization, the sperm's genetic information doesn't "kick in" until the embryo reaches the eight-cell stage of development. Until that time, the embryo only utilizes the stored genetic materials from the egg to develop. After the eight-cell stage, the embryo stops utilizing these materials, which gradually begin to decay, and begins to use its own genetic information (genome) to develop (this is known as genomic activation, or the maternal-to-zygotic transition [MZT]). This process requires multiple steps and the activation of a number of genes at specific times, and errors at any of these steps or timings can hinder early embryonic development. For example, if a gene for cell division is missing or not activated properly, the cells may not be able to divide. Further, if the egg's genetic materials do not decay at a normal pace, the MZT may not occur properly.
- **Genetic abnormalities**. Though this is a debated topic, some studies have found that embryos with genetic abnormalities (e.g., the wrong amount of DNA) often arrest early in development. These genetic

abnormalities can arise from the egg and/or sperm, or from errors in DNA replication at any stage of embryo development. Unfortunately, the chance of creating embryos with genetic abnormalities increases as women (and men, to a lesser extent) age, and embryos with genetic abnormalities are still able to develop normally (which is why PGT is often recommended). In fact, some studies have shown that embryos that develop and embryos that arrest have the same likelihood of having genetic abnormalities.

- **Errors in cell division.** If cell division is not occurring properly, the embryo will stop developing or will develop abnormally. For example, one cell may incorrectly divide into three cells, or DNA replication may occur within a cell even if cell division is not occurring (which would result in a cell with extra DNA).

- **Abnormal gene expression.** An embryo must activate (turn on) specific genes at precise times throughout its development. Failure to express these genes at the right times can impair development.

- **Mitochondrial impairment.** Mitochondria are small structures located inside every cell in our bodies. They supply cells with the energy that they need to function. Unsurprisingly, embryos contain a lot of mitochondria because they require a lot of energy to develop. Mitochondrial function can be impaired by aging and oxidative stress (the presence of too many reactive oxygen species in the body). When an embryo's mitochondrial function is impaired, it may not have enough energy to develop properly.

- **Sperm and/or egg quality issues.** Abnormalities in the quality of a sperm and/or egg can interfere with embryo development. For example, embryos created from sperm with fragmented DNA are less likely to develop into blastocysts than embryos created from sperm with non-fragmented DNA.

- **An abnormal shift in metabolism.** Early embryos require a lot of oxygen to obtain their energy. As they develop, they should shift to requiring less oxygen to obtain energy. If embryos fail to make this transition, their development may be impaired.

- **Abnormal protein synthesis (production).** Throughout embryonic development, structures known as RNA (ribonucleic acid) produce proteins that are essential for embryo development. If there are errors in the synthesis of any of these proteins, embryo development can be affected.

- **Suboptimal culture conditions.** This is uncommon, but it's possible that embryos in an IVF laboratory are exposed to suboptimal conditions, such as abnormal gas concentrations in the incubators or pollutants (volatile organic compounds, or VOCs) in the lab. These conditions can cause oxidative stress (an increase in the amount of reactive oxygen species, or ROS) and impair embryo development.

Embryo Grading/Morphology

All embryos have unique appearances even if they are at the same stage of development. Therefore, an embryo can be assessed (graded) based on its morphology, or physical appearance, to help predict its developmental potential.

There are standardized systems that many clinics use to grade embryos based on key physical characteristics, but some clinics may have unique grading systems. If your clinic grades embryos differently than described below, ask your care team to explain how their grading works.

While some IVF labs grade embryos on day 3 (3 days after insemination), many labs prefer to wait until day 5 to begin grading embryos. Some labs culture until day 7, while others do not.

Day 3 Grading

Day 3 embryos are known as cleavage-stage embryos (cleaving is another word for dividing), meaning that they should consist of multiple cells (blastomeres) as a result of cell division (mitosis). Though they consist of multiple cells, day 3 embryos are still the same size that they were on day 1, but their cells are smaller. Think of it like a birthday cake: the more slices you cut, the smaller each slice will be. Day 3 embryo grading normally consists of three criteria:[23]

- **The number of cells in the embryo.** It's normal for a day 3 embryo to consist of six to ten cells. Embryos with eight cells (Figure 7.12) have the highest live birth rates.

- **The percentage of fragmentation (blebbing) in the embryo.** Fragments are small pieces of the embryo's cells that break off as cell division occurs. Embryos with less than 20 percent fragmentation are associated with higher success rates than embryos with higher levels of fragmentation.

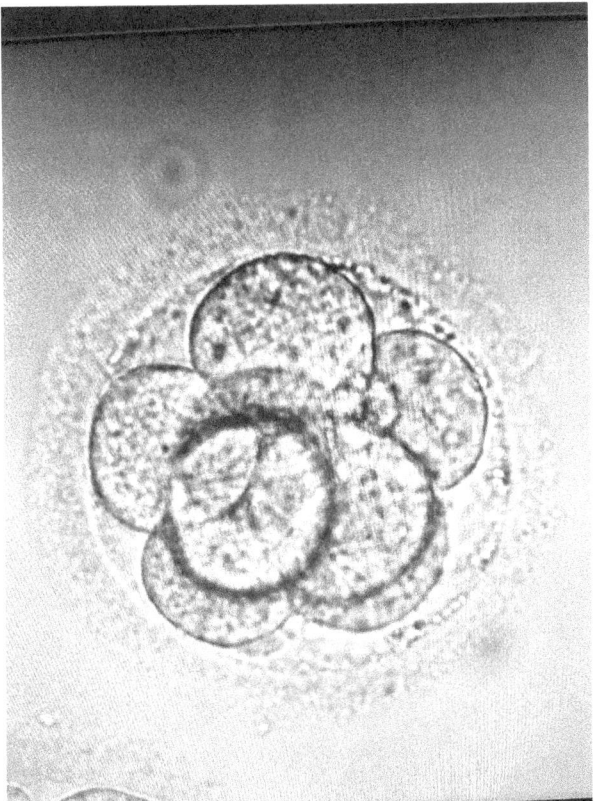

Figure 7.12 An eight-cell embryo on day 3 of development.

- **How symmetrical the cells in the embryo are.** As the number of cells in an embryo increases, the size of the cells decreases. And, since the cells in the embryo should all divide at roughly the same rate, they should all be perfectly or moderately symmetrical. Severe asymmetry may indicate that cell division is not occurring properly, which can interfere with embryonic development.

Some clinics may also grade a day 3 embryo's appearance using:

- A numerical scale ranging from 1–4 or 1–5, with 1 being the best
- An alphabetical scale ranging from A-C or A-D, with A being the best
- A good (G), fair (F), or poor (P) system

Some clinics may also include other criteria in their day 3 grades, such as the abnormal presence of:

- Multinucleation (cells with multiple nuclei in them)
- Vacuoles (fluid-filled spaces in the cells that are surrounded by membranes)
- Granules (small dark particles distinct from cellular fragments)

Do not get discouraged if your day 3 embryos are not within these ranges because they can still result in healthy live births, though their success rates are lower when compared to high-quality day 3 embryos.[24].

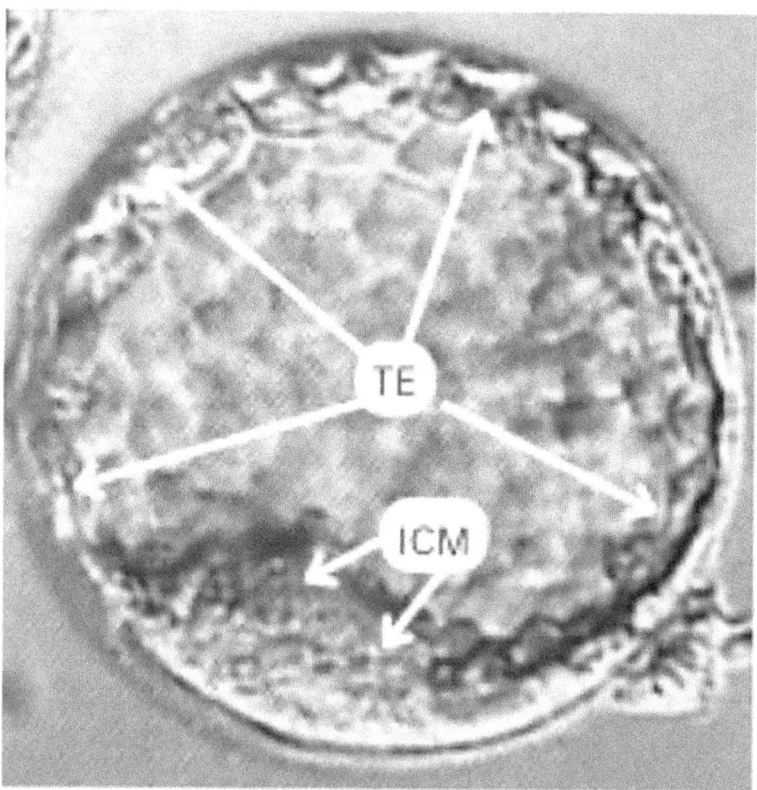

Figure 7.13 A blastocyst has two distinct cell lines: an inner cell mass (ICM) and trophectoderm (TE).

Day 5 (Blastocyst) Grading

Most clinics grade embryos on days 5 through 6 or 7 (depending on your clinic's protocol) once they reach the blastocyst stage of development (see table above). At this point, a cavity (blastocoel) and two distinct cell lines begin to form in the embryo (see Figure 7.13):

1. The inner cell mass (ICM) is a group of cells that can eventually develop into the fetus.
2. The trophectoderm epithelium (TE) cells form the outer layer of the embryo and can eventually develop into the placenta and other non-fetal tissues.

A common grading system is the Gardner scale (outlined in the table below), which which evaluates three key features:

- **The stage of development, (also called the degree of expansion)**, often recorded as a number or letter(s).
- **The appearance of the ICM**, often recorded as an A, B, or C (sometimes D, depending on your clinic's system), with A being the highest grade.
- **The appearance of the TE**, often recorded as an A, B, or C (sometimes D, depending on your clinic's system), with A being the highest grade.

Stage of Development/ Level of Expansion	ICM Grading Description	TE Grading Description
1 (early blastocyst, or EB): the blastocoel (cavity) is less than 50% of the volume of the embryo	A (good) = Very compact, many cells, well-defined	A (good) = Many uniform cells, few gaps or irregularities, well-developed
2 (blastocyst, B, or BL): the blastocoel is more than 50% of the volume of the embryo	B (fair) = Somewhat or loosely compact, average number of cells	B (fair) = Moderate number of cells that are mostly uniform, some gaps or abnormalities
3 (full blastocyst, or FB): the blastocoel completely fills the embryo		
4 (expanded blastocyst, XB, or ExB): the embryo's shell (zona pellucida) thins as the embryo's volume increases	C/D (poor) = Absent, not compact, very few cells, fragmented, degenerate	C/D (poor) = Absent, very few cells, many gaps or abnormalities, degenerate
5 (hatching blastocyst, or HgB): the embryo begins to emerge from an opening in the zona pellucida		
6 (hatched blastocyst, HB, or HdB): the embryo fully emerges from its zona pellucida		

Embryo Grading Examples

- An expanded blastocyst with a very compact ICM and average TE is a 4AB.
- A hatching blastocyst with a somewhat compact ICM and below-average TE is a 5BC.

Embryo Grading and Success Rates

High ("excellent" or "good") quality embryos have higher clinical pregnancy and live birth rates when compared to poor-quality embryos.[25,26] However, embryo grading is subjective, meaning that it may differ between embryologists, and an embryo's grade is only one factor to consider when predicting its chance of success. For example, an embryo's grade does not determine if its cells have the correct number of chromosomes.

Poor-Quality Embryos

Does all of this mean that poor-quality embryos are not worth transferring? Absolutely not. Poor-quality blastocysts can still result in healthy live births, especially when their cells have the right number of chromosomes. Though poor-quality embryos tend to yield lower implantation rates than high-quality embryos, poor-quality embryos that do implant have similar clinical pregnancy and live birth rates compared to high-quality embryos.[27] Keep in mind that some clinics will not transfer poor-quality embryos.

Embryo Transfers

An embryo transfer involves transferring an embryo(s) into the uterus of an intended parent or gestational carrier (surrogate).

There are many types of transfers that can be performed (see table below), and each clinic may have its own protocols before, during, and after each embryo transfer.

Common Types of Embryo Transfers	
Fresh	Frozen
Day 3 (Cleavage)	Day 5+ (Blastocyst)
Medicated (Artificial, Programmed)	Unmedicated (Natural)

Fresh Versus Frozen Embryo Transfers

Embryo transfers can occur during or after an IVF cycle.

Fresh embryo transfers are usually performed 3 or 5 days after eggs are retrieved (or thawed) and inseminated in the lab. This means that the embryo(s) was not frozen before the transfer occurred (though a transfer may also be considered "frozen" if the eggs were frozen prior to insemination). Fresh embryos transfers can lead to a pregnancy faster and reduce the risk of embryo damage during the freezing and thawing processes, but fresh embryo transfers result in increased incidences of preterm birth, low birth weight, and small-for-gestational-age outcomes compared to frozen embryo transfers.[28]

Frozen embryo transfers occur after an embryo(s) is frozen in an IVF cycle (i.e., in a later menstrual cycle). Frozen embryos undergo a warming (thawing) process (see below) a few hours before an embryo transfer is scheduled (timing varies between clinics).

Regardless, there are situations in which embryos must be frozen, including when:

- PGT is performed (it takes about two weeks to get these results back). An embryo can be biopsied and transferred on the same day, but the PGT results will not be available prior to the transfer.
- There is a risk of developing ovarian hyperstimulation syndrome (OHSS) and/or abnormal hormone levels following ovarian stimulation and the egg retrieval procedure.
- The uterine lining is not thick enough prior to the fresh transfer and it must be canceled.
- No embryos have fully developed at the time of the scheduled fresh transfer, so the transfer is canceled and the embryos are given another day (or two) to develop before being frozen.
- Extra embryos that are created during an IVF cycle are frozen and stored for future use.

There is some debate as to which option yields the best results. Some studies have found that frozen embryo transfers yield higher success rates than fresh transfers,[29] while others have found no significant differences between the two.[30,31,32]

Day 3 (Cleavage) Versus Day 5+ (Blastocyst) Transfers

Embryos can be transferred at any point in their development, though most clinics either transfer embryos at the cleavage stage (usually day 3) or blastocyst stage. Fresh blastocyst transfers usually occur on day 5 of an IVF cycle, while frozen blastocyst transfers can include embryos that were frozen on days 5, 6, or

7 in a previous IVF cycle. There are a number of pros and cons associated with day 3 versus blastocyst transfers[33,34,35] (see table below), so talk with your fertility specialist about which option is best for you.

Day 3 Transfers	
Pros	Cons
More embryos are often available for transfer on day 3 since some embryos do not continue to develop past day 3 in an IVF lab (see section above regarding embryo arrest), so placing these embryos into the uterus can give them their best chance of developing in a natural environment. This is often recommended when a small number of embryos are produced in an IVF cycle.	The transfer of a single day 3 embryo has lower implantation and live birth rates when compared to the transfer of a single day 5 embryo. Therefore, multiple day 3 embryos are often transferred to yield similar success rates to day 5 transfers of just one embryo, but the transfer of multiple day 3 embryos greatly increases the risk of multiple pregnancies (twins or more), which can cause pregnancy and neonatal complications.
Day 3 embryo transfers yield similar clinical and ongoing pregnancy rates compared to day 5 embryo transfers, though multiple day 3 embryos must be transferred compared to one day 5 embryo to yield these results.	Many embryos do not develop past day 3 whether they are in an incubator or uterus, so transferring an embryo on day 3 that will not develop can provide false hope and unnecessary anxiety.
	PGT is not routinely performed on day 3 embryos, so more embryos with genetic abnormalities are likely to be transferred.
	Day 3 embryos are still in the fallopian tube during an *in vivo* (in the body) pregnancy. Therefore, the uterus is not prepared for (synchronized with) the implantation of a day 3 embryo, so the embryo will spend a few days moving around in the uterus before implantation occurs.

Blastocyst Transfers	
Pros	Cons
Embryos have proved their viability in culture by this time since their development progressed from day 3 (in particular, they have completed the maternal-zygotic transition).	Some embryos do not develop past day 3, so it's more likely to have few (or no) embryos available for transfer on day 5 versus day 3.
Fewer embryos need to be transferred to yield acceptable success rates. In fact, only one embryo is transferred in the majority of blastocyst embryo transfers. This drastically reduces the risk of multiple pregnancies (twins, etc.).	Embryos remain in culture for a few more days as opposed to the natural environment of the uterus.
PGT can be performed on blastocyst embryos, which increases the chances of transferring a genetically normal embryo.	Some studies suggest that blastocyst embryo transfers increase the chances of an embryo splitting to produce twins, triplets, etc.
The uterus is prepared (synchronized) for embryo implantation shortly after a blastocyst transfer occurs.	

Medicated Versus Unmedicated Transfer Cycles

There are multiple ways to prepare the body for an embryo transfer. The two primary methods are medicated (artificial, or programmed) or unmedicated (natural) preparation, though partially medicated cycles also exist. Regardless of the type of transfer, it's important that the uterine lining is normal in appearance (trilaminar) and thick enough that an embryo can implant into it once the transfer has occurred. Keep in mind that the protocols, dosages, and types of medications used may differ between clinics.

Many studies have found no significant differences in success rates between medicated and natural transfers, while others claim that natural cycles have improved outcomes.[36,37] Talk with your doctor about which option is best for you.

Medicated frozen embryo transfer cycles. Many clinics prefer medicated frozen embryo transfers because they require less monitoring and the timing of the transfer can be controlled. However, medicated FET cycles are more expensive, and studies have found that they increase the risks of pregnancy-induced hypertension, preeclampsia, and postpartum hemorrhage.[38]

Timeline

Often, women will begin taking birth control pills (OCPs) and/or Lupron during the menstrual cycle *prior to* their FET cycles. These medications "quiet" the ovaries so eggs do not mature and ovulation does not occur. Once instructed, the OCPs and/or Lupron are stopped to induce menses (a period).

    A monitoring (ultrasound and bloodwork) appointment is usually scheduled a few days after your period begins to ensure that your uterine lining is thin and your reproductive hormone levels are at their baseline levels. If the monitoring results are normal, you may be instructed to begin administering estrogen as either a pill, injection, or patch. The goal of the estrogen is to thicken the uterine lining and prevent ovulation from occurring. Because ovulation does not occur, a corpus luteum (the structure in the ovaries that produces progesterone following ovulation) does not form.

    Roughly two weeks later, another monitoring appointment is scheduled to determine if your uterine lining displays a trilaminar (three distinct layers) pattern and has thickened from the estrogen, which signify that the lining is properly preparing for embryo implantation. Your reproductive hormone levels may also be measured via a blood test. If your lining is insufficient, your estrogen dosage may need to be increased and/or your transfer may need to be postponed or canceled. If your monitoring results are normal, you may be instructed to begin administering progesterone along with estrogen. Progesterone is typically administered as an injection (PIO), vaginal suppository, and/or pill. The purpose of progesterone is to cause the uterine lining to continue thickening and support the pregnancy if implantation occurs. This would normally be accomplished by the corpus luteum following ovulation, but the corpus luteum is not formed during medicated cycles, so exogenous progesterone is required.

    Some clinics also prescribe an antibiotic and/or steroid on the same day as progesterone administration. Depending on the protocol, these may be continued for a few days leading up to the transfer.

    Blastocyst embryo transfers are typically scheduled on the sixth day of progesterone administration, and day 3 transfers are scheduled on the fourth day of progesterone administration. Additional monitoring may also be required a few days prior to your transfer.

    E2 and progesterone are administered until a pregnancy test is completed. If pregnancy occurs, estrogen and progesterone are administered for eight to twelve weeks (or until you are instructed to stop), which is when the placenta takes over estrogen and progesterone production to maintain the pregnancy. If a pregnancy does not occur, estrogen and progesterone administration are discontinued to induce menses.

Medicated fresh embryo transfer. For a fresh embryo transfer, progesterone is administered daily beginning on the night of your egg retrieval. An antibiotic and/or steroid regimen may be prescribed for the following day, which is continued until the day of the transfer.

Bloodwork and an ultrasound are often completed before the transfer to ensure that the endometrium has thickened enough for the transfer to occur. Progesterone administration is continued until a pregnancy test is completed. If pregnancy occurs, progesterone is administered for eight to twelve weeks (or until instructed to stop). If pregnancy does not occur, progesterone administration is discontinued to induce menses.

Unmedicated embryo transfer cycles rely on your body's hormones to thicken the uterine lining in preparation for embryo implantation rather than medications. One key difference is that ovulation *does* occur during these cycles, which must be closely monitored. While fresh embryo transfers are more cost-effective and do not require medications, they are not recommended for those with ovulatory dysfunctions and require more monitoring than medicated FET cycles.

Timeline

At the start of your menstrual cycle in which the transfer will occur, a baseline monitoring (an ultrasound and bloodwork) appointment is scheduled a few days after your period starts. If these monitoring results are normal, you must begin to track your ovulation. When your LH surge occurs (which indicates that ovulation is about to occur), you should alert your clinic. Leading up to ovulation, you will likely require frequent monitoring (usually an ultrasound and/or blood work) at your clinic to confirm when ovulation occurs. Your clinic will also observe your uterine lining to ensure that it is thickening leading up to ovulation.

Of note, some clinics prescribe the medication Letrozole for the first five days of your cycle to help control the timing of ovulation. Alternatively, an hCG injection can be administered, which triggers ovulation to occur thirty-six to forty hours later.

Once ovulation has been confirmed and your uterine lining is thickened, your embryo transfer can be scheduled a few days later. In some situations, progesterone is administered daily beginning the day after this appointment and should be continued until you are instructed to stop. In other situations, progesterone is not administered. You may also need to complete additional monitoring before proceeding with the transfer.

Assisted Hatching

For an embryo to implant into the uterine lining, it must hatch from its shell (zona pellucida). While most embryos naturally hatch on their own, some embryos may not due to intrinsic (internal) errors in the embryo or shel structure. Most clinics routinely perform assisted hatching (AH) on embryos to ensure that they are able to hatch from their shells once they are transferred.

The most common method for AH is to create a small hole in the shell using a laser. An embryo's cells should not be harmed in this process. AH can be performed at any time in an IVF cycle, but it's most commonly performed on day 3, before an embryo is biopsied, or before an embryo transfer. Embryos that are hatching on their own do not require AH.

Surprisingly, most (but not all) studies have not found improved clinical pregnancy or live birth rates when AH is performed on embryos. Further, multiple studies have found an increased risk of monozygotic twinning (developing twins from the same embryo) when AH is performed, though this data does not definitively conclude that the increased risk of monozygotic twinning is a direct result of AH.[39]

Regardless, AH is still routinely performed in most IVF labs since it ensures that an embryo can overcome any abnormalities that interfere with hatching and implantation. For example, an embryo with an abnormally thick or hardened shell may not be able to hatch on its own and implant into the uterine lining.

Hyaluronan-Enriched Transfer Medium for Embryo Transfers

Hyaluronan-enriched transfer media (HETM) such as EmbryoGlue® are commercially available products that contain hyaluronan and albumin and are sometimes utilized for embryo transfers. Hyaluronan and albumin are naturally produced in the female reproductive tract and support embryo adhesion (the ability to stick to the uterine lining) and implantation. Embryos are placed into HETM for a few moments before an embryo transfer and are transferred into the uterus in a small volume of HETM. Most studies have found improved implantation and live birth rates with the use of HETM, especially after previously failed embryo transfers, but these studies are limited and more research is required. Studies have also found an increased risk of multiple pregnancies (twins or more) when HETM are used, though this cannot be directly attributed to the use of HETM.[40,41] Regardless, HETM may be recommended in cases of

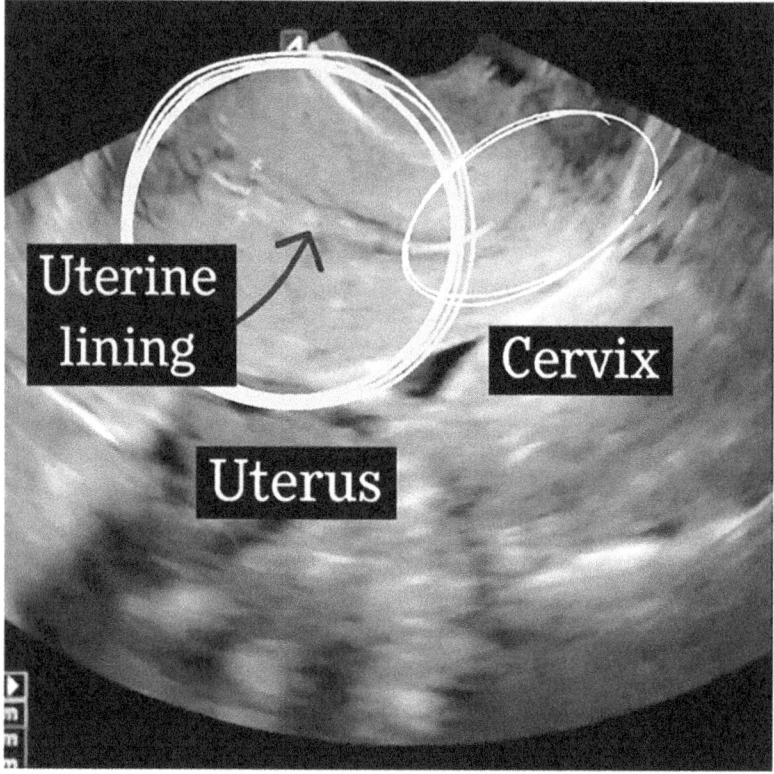

Figure 7.14 An ultrasound view of the cervix, uterus, and uterine lining (endometrium).

recurrent implantation failure (repetitive failed implantation following the transfer of high-quality embryos).

Trial Transfers

A trial (mock) embryo is a practice procedure that mimics an actual embryo transfer. It can be performed at any time prior to the real transfer, though it is often performed during another procedure, such as a hysteroscopy or uterine biopsy, for convenience. Many clinics require these procedures because they determine if the uterus is positioned normally, ensure that the transfer catheter has a pathway into the uterus, and help determine the size of the catheter that is needed at the time of transfer.

Trial transfers are minimally invasive and usually take about five to ten minutes to complete. The procedure should be relatively painless, though mild cramping has been reported.

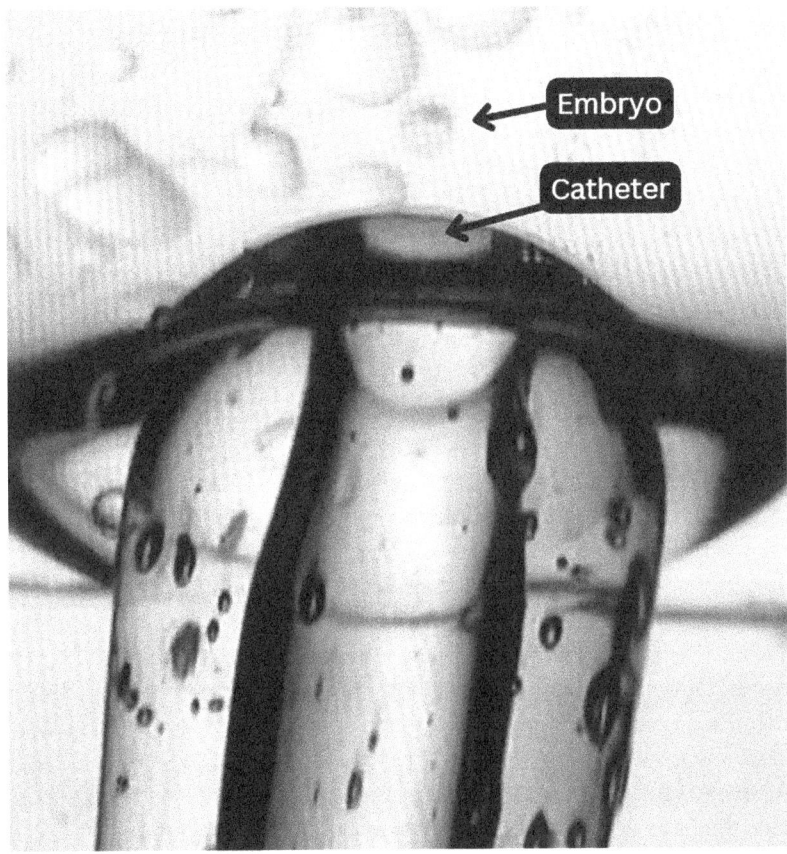

Figure 7.15 An embryo entering a catheter during an embryo transfer procedure.

Preparing for an Embryo Transfer

Aside from properly administering your transfer medications (if needed) and attending your scheduled monitoring appointments, there is not much preparation required for an embryo transfer. However, you should always follow any instructions provided by your IVF clinic staff.

On the day of your embryo transfer, you will check in and be escorted to a private area to change. Try to have a full bladder prior to your transfer since this provides a straighter path for the catheter and improves ultrasound visualization. You will then be escorted to the operating room and will be seated on an exam table. Your identity will be confirmed, and you may even receive a picture of your embryo(s) to take home.

The Embryo Transfer Procedure

Most embryo transfers are not performed under sedation, though there are exceptions. The procedure is minimally invasive and takes roughly five to fifteen minutes to complete. During the procedure, you will lie on your back with your feet in stirrups.

A fertility specialist will insert a speculum into your vagina to visualize and clean your cervix (the lower portion of your uterus). Some of this fluid may leak from the vagina after the procedure, but this fluid does not contain the embryo. An abdominal ultrasound is used to view the uterus and cervix throughout the process (Figure 7.14).

A thin catheter is then inserted through the cervix and into the uterus. Transfer catheters actually contain a plastic external sheath and thin flexible inner catheter. In some clinics, the embryo is already loaded into this inner catheter. In these situations, the embryo (and some fluid) is injected into the uterus once it is in the correct position.

In other clinics, the external sheath acts as a guide for the catheter that contains the embryo. Once the external sheath is in place, the inner catheter is removed. The embryo is then loaded into the inner catheter (Figure 7.15), which is thread through the external sheath into the uterus. Once the tip of the inner catheter is in position on the ultrasound monitor, the embryo (and some fluid) is injected into the uterus.

Afterward, the catheter is removed and inspected under a microscope to ensure that the embryo was successfully transferred into the uterus. If the embryo is retained in the catheter, it is reloaded and the process is repeated (this has not been shown to affect success rates).[42]

After the Transfer

You do not have to remain at your clinic after your transfer, though some clinics recommend that you rest for a few minutes afterward. Unless instructed otherwise, it's okay for you to drive home as soon as the transfer is over. Before you leave, your fertility specialist should review your rules and restrictions for the next few days. Always follow these rules and restrictions, and contact your clinic if you have any questions about certain activities before performing them. In general, it's recommended that you:

- Avoid strenuous exercise and heavy lifting
- Move around (bed rest is typically not recommended)

- Avoid hot tubs/jacuzzis and anything else that can elevate your body temperature
- Maintain a healthy diet and stay hydrated
- Avoid smoking, alcohol consumption, and exposure to harmful chemicals and toxins

After the embryo is transferred, it will move around the uterus for twenty-four to forty-eight hours (or longer if it's a day 3 embryo) as it continues developing. It will also hatch from its shell if it hasn't already. After this time, the embryo will hopefully implant into the uterine lining. If implantation occurs and the embryo continues developing, cells in its placenta begin to produce the hormone hCG (human chorionic gonadotropin). As the placenta develops, the amount of hCG production increases. hCG travels through the body and can be detected in the blood or urine.

A clinical (quantitative) blood test is typically scheduled 9–12 days after an embryo transfer occurs. This test measures the level of hCG in the blood, which indicates whether or not embryo implantation has occurred. Normally, hCG levels >5 mIU/mL are considered positive, but it's important that these levels continue to double every forty-eight to seventy-two hours. Many clinics require one or two additional blood tests to ensure that your levels are rising appropriately. If your blood test is negative, you will stop taking your medications, which should induce menses (your period).

Unfortunately, some embryo transfers are unsuccessful, meaning that they do not result in healthy live births. Please refer to Chapter 9 for information about failed embryo transfers.

Embryo Splitting

Studies have shown a higher incidence of monozygotic twinning (one embryo splits to form twins), or MZT, in IVF pregnancies compared to spontaneous conceptions. MZT is associated with increased pregnancy and neonatal complications, including intrauterine growth restriction (delayed growth in utero), preterm delivery, low birth weight, and neonatal morbidity and mortality. Therefore, IVF clinics have increased the number of single-embryo transfers (the transfer of one embryo) to alleviate the risk of multiple gestations (twins or more).

It's unknown exactly what causes the increased incidence of MZT following IVF, but some theories are that it is caused by:[43,44]

- ICSI (controversial data)
- Biopsying the embryo for PGT

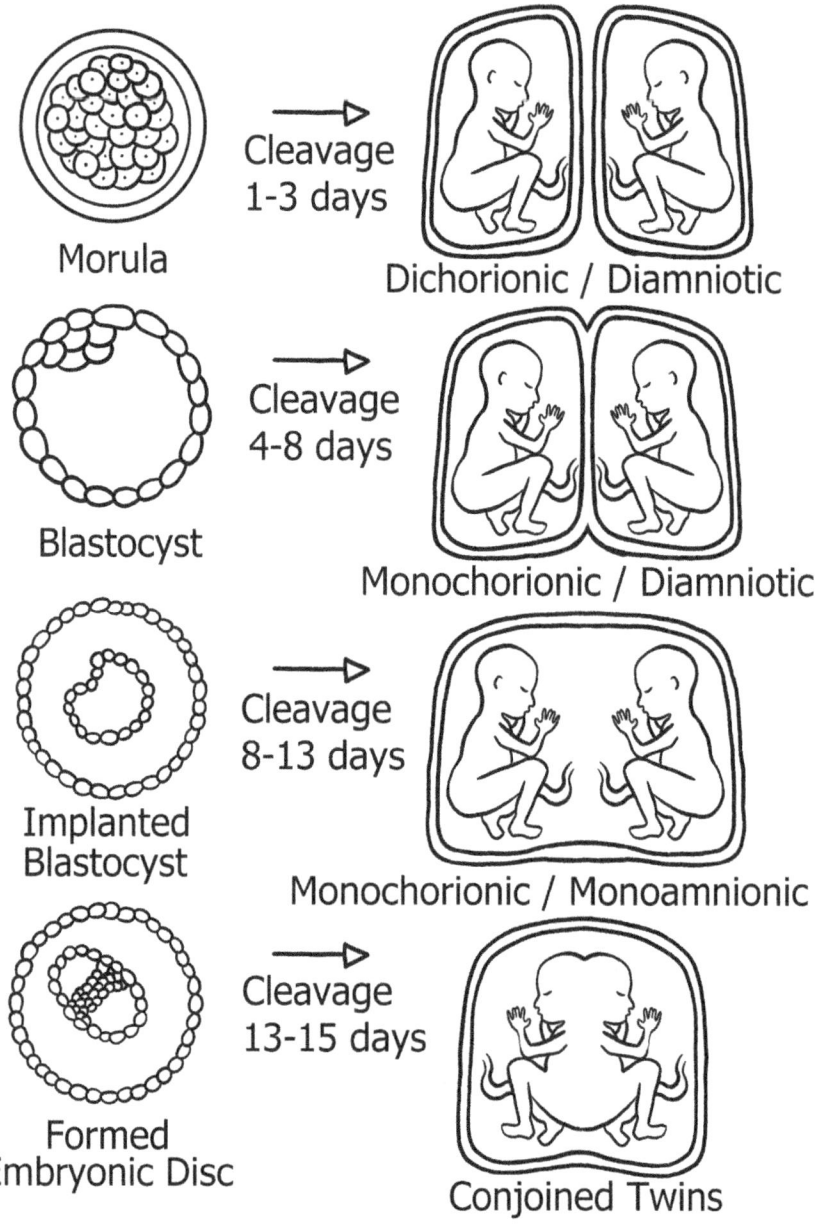

Figure 7.16 Embryo splitting can occur at various times during early embryonic development.

- Assisted hatching
- Embryo freezing and thawing prior to transfer (controversial data)
- Prolonged embryo culture

Unfortunately, there is almost never a way to determine if an embryo will split before it is transferred. In some cases, it may be possible to observe two inner cell masses (ICMs) in an embryo, which could both develop into fetuses. However, this is rare and still does not guarantee that an embryo will split after it is transferred.

Embryo splitting can occur at any time before or after implantation, and the timing of the splitting determines if the twins will share a placenta and/or amniotic sac in utero (Figure 7.16).

How Many Embryos Should be Transferred?

An IVF cycle is considered successful when it results in a healthy live birth, though the goal of an IVF cycle is the birth of one (singleton) healthy baby. Years ago, it was common for IVF clinics to transfer multiple embryos at one time to optimize success rates. However, only one (sometimes two) embryos are now routinely transferred at a time to yield similar success rates due to improved technologies and culture conditions. Typically, two day 3 (D3) embryos or one blastocyst (day 5, 6, or 7) embryo are transferred at a time.

The transfer of multiple embryos increases the incidence of multiple gestations (twins, triplets, etc.). Further, there is a risk of embryos splitting, which can also result in a multiple gestation (see section above). Numerous studies have found that multiple gestations are at an increased risk of pregnancy and neonatal (after birth) complications (especially premature delivery), with the severity of complications increasing with the number of fetuses (i.e., quadruplets are at a higher risk than twins). Multiple gestations can also create financial burdens that arise from additional hospital costs, supplies (bottles, diapers, etc.), and childcare.

The 2021 American Society for Reproductive Medicine (ASRM) guidelines state the following for good prognosis patients:[45]

- "Transfer of a euploid embryo should be limited to one, regardless of patient age.
- Patients <35 years of age should be strongly encouraged to receive a single-embryo transfer, regardless of the embryo stage.

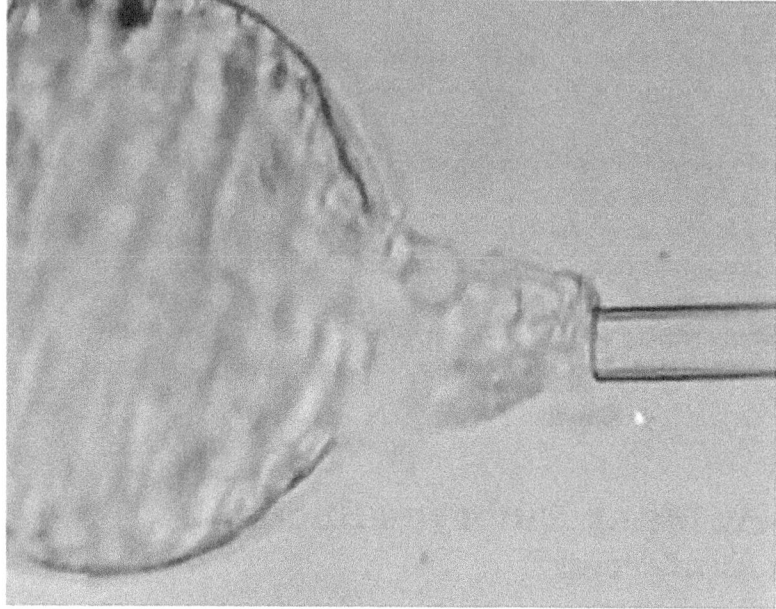

Figure 7.17 During the embryo biopsy procedure, a few cells are removed from the embryo's trophectoderm for preimplantation genetic testing (PGT).

- For patients between 35 and 37 years of age, strong consideration should be made for a single-embryo transfer.
- For patients between 38 and 40 years of age, no more than 3 untested cleavage-stage embryos or 2 blastocysts should be transferred.
- Patients 41–42 years of age should plan to receive no more than 4 untested cleavage-stage embryos or 3 blastocysts."

If your IVF cycle results in multiple gestation, you may have the option to reduce the number of fetuses through a process known as multifetal pregnancy reduction. This procedure can reduce the number of fetuses inside the womb, but it can also harm the remaining fetus and may have adverse psychological effects. This is not always possible, but you can talk with your doctor for more information if this applies to you.[46]

In some cases, a pregnancy may begin with twins but result in the loss of one of the twins. This is known as vanishing twin syndrome and unfortunately cannot be prevented.

Preimplantation Genetic Testing (PGT)

Preimplantation genetic testing (PGT) is a screening tool used to identify certain genetic abnormalities in embryos with over 95 percent accuracy. For more information about PGT results, see Chapter 8.

PGT is normally performed on embryos that have reached the blastocyst stages of development. PGT requires an embryo biopsy, during which approximately five cells are carefully removed from an embryo's trophectoderm (outer layer of cells that develop into the placenta) using a laser (Figure 7.17). Assisted hatching of the embryo's shell (zona pellucida) may need to be performed to access the embryo's cells inside its shell. The embryo is frozen at your IVF clinic and remains stored there in liquid nitrogen, while the biopsied sample is sent to a genetic testing facility. The biopsied samples remain frozen until they arrive at the genetic testing facility.

The genetic testing facility amplifies (makes many copies of) the DNA inside the cells within a biopsy sample. The DNA is then analyzed and a report is sent to your IVF clinic. This report should indicate whether or not each tested embryo is suitable for transfer.

In general, over 95 percent of embryos survive the biopsy procedure. However, an embryo with a below-average trophectoderm may be affected by the biopsy procedure since approximately five cells are removed from it. This leaves behind very few trophectoderm cells, which are important for embryo implantation. Further, poor-quality embryos are less likely to survive the freezing and thawing processes (see below). In rare cases, mechanical errors during a biopsy procedure can damage an embryo, though these should be documented by your IVF lab staff.

It's possible to perform PGT on an embryo that has already been frozen. This process involves thawing, biopsying, and re-freezing the embryo. The biopsied sample is sent to a genetic testing facility for analysis, while the embryo remains frozen in the IVF lab. This is the same procedure that would occur if an already-tested embryo needs to be biopsied again (e.g., when there is not enough DNA present in the original biopsy sample to generate a result). There is a slight risk of damage to the embryo during these processes due to the additional mechanical manipulation involved, but most embryos (>90 percent) survive these procedures.

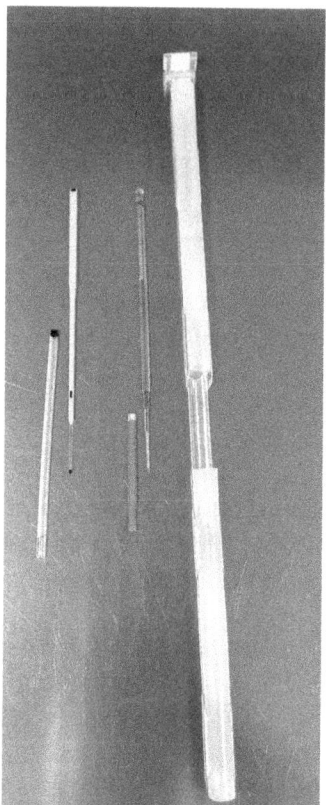

Figure 7.18 Embryos and eggs are often frozen on these or similar devices (left). The devices are stored in a plastic goblet that is attached to a metal cane with a labeled metal tag at the top (right).

Embryo Freezing

Embryo freezing (vitrification or flash freezing) is a technique that is performed in nearly every IVF clinic (it replaced the older method of slow freezing). This procedure normally consists of the following steps, though each lab may have its own protocols and devices:

1. The embryo(s) is placed into media (fluids) that contain high concentrations of substances known as cryoprotectant agents (CPAs). There are two types of CPAs: permeating CPAs that enter the cells to balance osmotic pressure, and non-permeating CPAs that remain outside the cells and help draw water out of them. They are often both used for embryo freezing. CPAs protect the embryo as it is frozen by:[47]

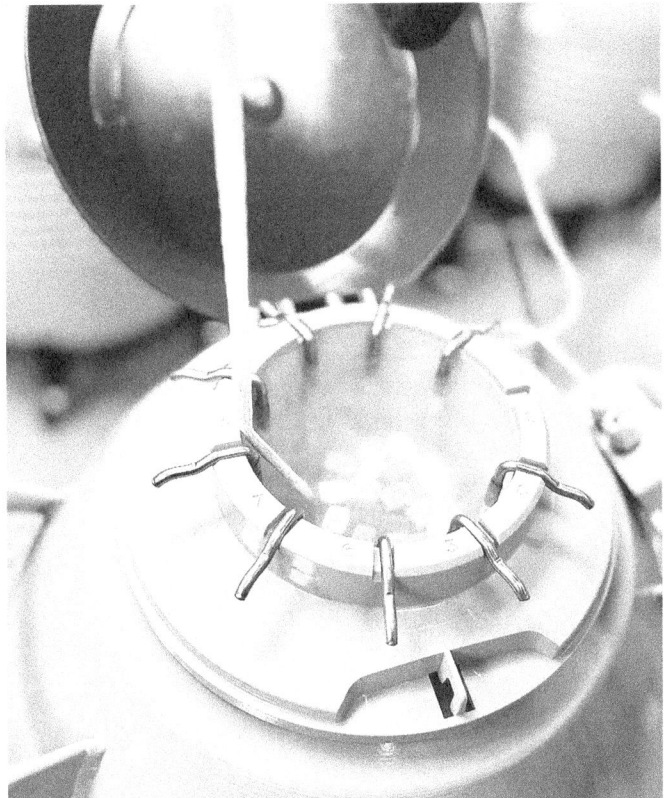

Figure 7.19 Frozen embryos, eggs, and sperm reside in dewars (cryotanks) that are routinely monitored and filled with liquid nitrogen.

    a. Gradually removing water from the embryo's cells to prevent ice crystal formation (ice crystals can damage the cells during freezing). Embryos normally collapse as water is removed from their cells. Some labs also manually collapse embryos before they're frozen. This means that a small laser pulse is applied between two cells in the embryo, which causes water to flow out of the embryo. This has been shown to improve survival rates since it removes excess water from the embryo, minimizing ice crystal formation. Permeable CPAs can then enter the cells as water is removed from them.

    b. Maintaining a low salt concentration in the embryo's cells (high concentrations can damage the cells).

2. The embryo(s) is placed on a "vitrification device," which typically consists of a transparent film (where the embryo is placed) and a plastic

handle for easy maneuvering. This device should contain a label with pertinent identifying information (your name, medical record number, etc.).

3. The device is quickly plunged into liquid nitrogen, which remains around −196°C. This rapid plunging prevents ice crystals from forming in the embryo and transforms the cells into a solid, glass-like state.

4. Each device is then securely closed and placed into a plastic goblet (cup) that is secured to a metal cane (Figure 7.18). The top of each cane should also be labeled for easy identification.

5. The metal cane is placed in a storage tank (called a cryotank or Dewar), which should be consistently monitored and refilled with liquid nitrogen to maintain proper conditions. (Figure 7.19).

Embryos can remain stored in liquid nitrogen indefinitely, during which time their cellular activity is halted (no development occurs). In fact, a healthy baby was recently born from an embryo that was frozen in 1994.

There are many reasons why embryos are frozen, including:

- Multiple embryos are produced during an IVF cycle that cannot be transferred during the cycle
- A high risk for the development of OHSS (ovarian hyperstimulation syndrome) following an egg retrieval
- Abnormal hormone levels prior to or on the day of the embryo transfer, which might cause the transfer to be canceled
- The embryo is biopsied for PGT (it can take roughly two weeks to obtain PGT results)
- A person/couple wishes to preserve embryos for future use (fertility preservation or embryo banking) or donation to another person/couple
- Other personal or medical reasons, such as upcoming chemotherapy.

Embryos can be frozen at any time in their development, and there do not appear to be differences in the survival rates when embryos are frozen on day 3 versus at the blastocyst stage of development. Overall, less than 5 percent of embryos do not survive the freezing and thawing processes (this means that less than half of the embryo is alive post-thaw). Failed survival is most common with poor-quality embryos (those with fewer cells than average or those that took longer to develop).[48]

Embryo Warming ("Thawing")

Warming ("thawing") embryos is essentially the opposite process of freezing them, during which embryos are:

1. Quickly removed from liquid nitrogen (LN2) and placed into a thawing solution
2. Moved through one or more drops of media that remove the cryoprotectant agent and add water back into the embryo's cells
3. Placed into a warm culture medium inside a sterile dish, which remains in an incubator

This process causes the embryo's cells to re-expand, though full re-expansion can take a few hours to complete. Studies have found that embryos are more likely to yield high success rates when they:[49,50]

- Re-expand at a normal rate following the thaw (usually within two to four hours)
- Display little to no cellular damage after they are thawed
- Were frozen as high-quality embryos
- Maintain their quality after they are thawed
- Remain intact after they are thawed

Embryos are normally thawed a few hours prior to an embryo transfer, and the elapsed time does not seem to affect the success rates of the transfer. Embryos should resume their development after they are thawed.

It's common for some of an embryo's cells to not survive the freezing/thawing procedures, though usually more than 50 percent of the cells do survive. However, some embryos may not survive due to:[51]

- The embryo's plasma membrane doesn't allow for the proper removal of water and/or the uptake of enough cryoprotectant to protect the embryo's cells during freezing. Or the plasma membrane doesn't allow for proper reuptake of water and/or removal of cryoprotectant during thawing. Cryoprotectants are actually toxic to embryos if they are handled incorrectly. Therefore, it's important that they are removed in a timely manner before they can damage the embryo's cells. There must also be a gradual removal of water from the embryo's cells since rapid pressure changes can damage the cells. If enough water is not removed, ice crystals can form during freezing and damage the embryo's cells.

- Certain errors in an embryo's genetic makeup can interfere with normal freezing/thawing
- Embryos that are frozen with fewer than average cells have a higher likelihood of more than 50 percent of the cells not surviving
- Errors in cryopreservation (e.g., leaving the embryo in media too long) or storage tank malfunctions (this is rare because storage tanks should consistently be monitored).

Note: the process of freezing/thawing eggs (oocytes) is very similar to that of embryos. However, variations in protocols may differ between labs.

Embryo Disposition

Before you begin IVF, you will likely sign consents stating whether or not you would like to freeze (cryopreserve) extra embryos that may be created during your IVF cycle. Most people elect to freeze extra embryos in case multiple embryo transfers are required or multiple children are desired. In addition to this option, you should select how you would like any of your frozen embryos disposed of in the event of death of one or both partners. Note that these options may differ between countries and clinics based on laws and policies. Common options include:

- Transferring ownership to the surviving partner, if applicable
- Discarding the embryos
- Donating the embryos to research
- Transferring ownership of the embryos to another person (this usually requires additional legal documentation)

Additionally, you will likely sign a consent stating whether or not you want your embryos to undergo preimplantation genetic testing (PGT). If you elect to perform PGT on your embryos, you may also need to designate how you wish to dispose of embryos that are deemed chromosomally abnormal (aneuploid) or unsuitable for transfer. Common options include discarding the embryos or donating them to research.

If you complete an IVF cycle and have extra frozen embryos, you will likely be required to pay a monthly or yearly storage fee to keep your embryos frozen. Most clinics will either keep your embryos frozen at the clinic or will transport them to an outside storage facility. However, if you are no longer undergoing fertility treatment, you may have the option to sign a consent at any time stating what you wish to do with your frozen embryos. This is often an emotionally challenging decision which requires careful consideration.

Though each clinic may have its own options, there are generally five options regarding the fate of extra embryos. Note that these options may also not be available in all clinics due to laws and policies:

1. **Discard them.** In these situations, the embryos are gently removed from liquid nitrogen (on their vitrification devices). Instead of being placed in a culture medium to promote development, the embryos are allowed to thaw and gradually reach room temperature on their devices. This prevents any further development of the embryos. The embryos are then placed in a biohazard container. Alternatively, you may choose to take the discarded embryos and dispose of them in your own manner (e.g., a burial).

2. **Donate them to research.** Some clinics allow you to donate embryos to research, in which case they will ultimately be discarded. There are laws in place regarding the use of donated embryos, so they will never be transferred to another person's uterus. Research embryos are normally used to train new embryologists and complete research projects within the IVF lab. If your clinic does not allow you to donate embryos to research but you would like to, consider contacting other clinics that may accept your embryos for research purposes.

3. **Donate them to another person/couple.** Though this process is a bit lengthier than the other options, embryo donation to another person/couple has become a popular option for unused embryos. While some clinics have in-house embryo donation programs, you may also choose to donate them to an outside agency (see Chapter 12 for more information about embryo donation and adoption).

4. **Keep them in storage.** If you are not ready to discard or donate your embryos, you have the option to keep them in storage, though you will likely need to continue paying a storage fee for these embryos and/or have the embryos sent to an outside storage facility.

5. **A compassionate transfer.** This process involves transferring your remaining embryos to your uterus at a time in your menstrual cycle that you are least likely to get pregnant (e.g., right after your period begins). Not all clinics offer compassionate transfers.

Karli's Story

After five years off birth control and one year of testing and trying with no results, my husband and I decided to seek help. Just making the consultation appointment gave me hope and then, after we decided to proceed with IVF, a pregnancy and baby couldn't come soon enough. After completing all the tests, I found out that I would need to have surgery to remove uterine polyps and that I had very low AMH, which meant that I would likely have a low number of eggs retrieved. Following my surgery, I had recurrent ovarian cysts for four months and had to keep pushing back my egg retrieval. After we finally completed an IVF cycle with PGT testing, we ended up with one viable embryo.

Through every result and every hurdle, I took to Google for information and here is what I can tell you:

- *No journey and body are the same or will respond the same.*
- *Comparing yourself to others will kill your joy and cause you unnecessary stress.*
- *Just because your path is taking longer than expected doesn't mean it won't happen for you.*
- *There will be highs and lows during your journey.*
- *Don't suffer in silence. Find a few people who you can confide in, be honest with your partner, share when you are scared or suffering, be selfish with your time, and put self-care above everything when you can.*
- *If you are confused about anything during your process, call your clinic instead of relying on Google or another person who did IVF.*

Following the transfer of our one embryo, I limited social media, said "no" to things that would cause me stress, relaxed way more than I needed to, and stayed hopeful. According to Google, the (very subjective) grade of my embryo had less than favorable success rates. But I am currently twelve weeks pregnant with our "one."

I hope that my story can give people hope. I had never been pregnant, didn't know I could get pregnant, and had a lot of obstacles to overcome. But I still had a successful result. I think so many women going through IVF focus on the numbers and others' unsuccessful stories, which can have a negative effect on their psyches.

I also think it's so important to tell yourself that every story is different, you could be the small percent that experiences success despite the odds, and that you are going to control what you can and release everything else to the Lord, universe, or anything else that you believe in.

Conclusions

IVF is a complex process with multiple variations. Your fertility specialist will help determine which treatment options are best for you.

Chapter 8
Preimplantation Genetic Testing (PGT)

The information in this chapter was contributed by Meaghan Doyle, MS, CGC, a certified genetic counselor specializing in fertility genetics and founder of DNAide Genetic Counselling.

Within the nucleus of every cell in our bodies are tightly packed structures called chromosomes that contain our genetic information, or DNA. DNA is organized into segments called genes, each of which provides instructions for how a pregnancy should form, how the body is built, and how the body functions.

Our DNA is tightly packed into structures called chromosomes so all of our DNA (there is a lot of it!) can fit into our cells. There are twenty-four different types of chromosomes in total:

- The first twenty-two chromosomes, called autosomes, are the same between most people. They carry the vast majority of our genetic information and determine our non-sexual traits (e.g., eye color, height, organ development). The autosomes are numbered from 1 to 22, generally according to their size (largest to smallest), though chromosome 21 is actually shorter than chromosome 22.
- The final two chromosomes are the sex chromosomes, X and Y. These chromosomes determine an individual's biological sex. Most people either have two X chromosomes (XX) or one X chromosome and one Y chromosome (XY), though rare variations exist. Individuals with XX sex chromosomes are typically born with female external genitalia and are assigned female at birth, while individuals with XY sex chromosomes are typically born with male external genitalia and assigned male at birth.

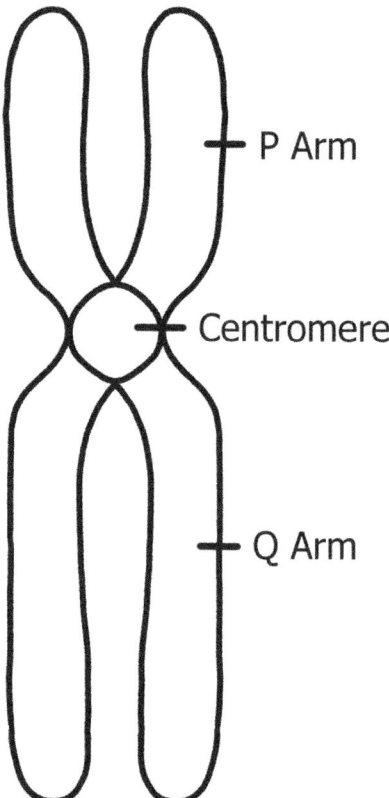

Figure 8.1 Chromosomes consist of P and Q arms with a central centromere.

All of our chromosomes come in pairs. We inherited one pair from the egg and the other from the sperm that created us. Most people have twenty-three pairs of chromosomes (twenty-two pairs of autosomes and one pair of sex chromosomes for a total of forty-six chromosomes in total) in each of their cells excluding egg and sperm cells. Since genes are the instructions for building and operating the human body, you can think of chromosomes like the instruction books for a developing pregnancy and baby.

Chromosomes have a specific structure composed of two "arms." The shorter arm is called the "p" arm. The other arm is longer and is called the "q" arm. The p and q arms of a chromosome are joined at a central region called the centromere (Figure 8.1). Specific sections on each arm are referred to as "bands," which help identify regions of interest on a chromosome. For example, p11.1 and q23.1 would be different bands of a chromosome. These banding patterns are used in genetic testing and diagnostics to pinpoint structural changes or abnormalities in chromosomes.

Preimplantation Genetic Testing

Preimplantation Genetic Testing (PGT) refers to genetic screening performed on an embryo before it is transferred into the uterus and implantation occurs. PGT requires an embryo biopsy, during which a few cells are removed from the embryo in an IVF lab (see Chapter 7). The biopsied samples are sent to a specialized PGT lab that analyzes the genetic material within these cells. While additional types of PGT may emerge in the future, there are currently three primary types, each serving a distinct purpose:

1. **Preimplantation Genetic Testing for Aneuploidy (PGT-A)** is the most commonly performed type of PGT. It screens embryos for chromosomal abnormalities (aneuploidies). For example, it can determine if an embryo has an entire extra chromosome (Trisomy 21 is a common example) or is missing part of a chromosome. Embryos with aneuploidy often fail to implant, result in miscarriage, or lead to the birth of a child with a genetic condition (a common example is Down syndrome). As long as your IVF clinic is capable of performing an embryo biopsy procedure (see Chapter 7), PGT-A is available to anyone undergoing IVF. Because of its complexity and clinical relevance, PGT-A is the focus of this chapter.

2. **Preimplantation Genetic Testing for Structural Rearrangements (PGT-SR)** is offered to individuals who are trying to conceive and have a known chromosome structural rearrangement, such as a translocation (a segment of one chromosome breaks off and attaches to a different chromosome) or inversion (a segment of a chromosome breaks off, rotates 180 degrees, and reattaches to the same chromosome in the reverse direction). These rearrangements increase the risk of creating embryos with aneuploidy. PGT-SR is similar to PGT-A but allows the PGT lab to detect specific chromosomal differences related to the known structural rearrangement in the person trying to conceive. PGT-SR can only be offered when the structural rearrangement is identified *prior* to embryo testing. It is often performed in conjunction with PGT-A to detect both inherited and random chromosomal abnormalities.

Adele's Story

Members of my husband's family have been diagnosed with a balanced translocation, so my husband was tested and it was confirmed that he also carried a balanced translocation on chromosomes eleven and twelve. This means that a piece of his eleventh chromosome broke off and attached to the twelfth chromosome, and a piece of his twelfth chromosome broke off and attached to the eleventh chromosome. People with balanced translocations are usually not harmed by these chromosomal rearrangements because they still have the right amount of DNA present for normal functioning. However, any offspring created from these individuals can have unbalanced translocations, which can be harmful or even fatal.

After this diagnosis, we were referred to a fertility center to discuss our options with a genetic fertility consultant and genetic counselor. They provided us with the option of IVF with preimplantation genetic testing (PGT), or natural conception (with the risk of early miscarriage) with testing via amniocentesis if the pregnancy continued to sixteen weeks.

With my husband's diagnosis, we were entitled to three funded cycles of IVF on the NHS (UK). We began our first cycle in March 2019 and had two genetically healthy embryos from this cycle. We later had each of these transferred (individually), which were both unsuccessful. In between these two embryo transfers, we also conceived naturally and had a miscarriage (likely due to the translocation).

Following the unsuccessful embryo transfers, our consultant recommended a hysteroscopy, which did not find any issues or concerns. We hadn't lost hope and continued on to our second IVF cycle.

We ended up with one genetically normal embryo, which was later transferred and (again) unsuccessful. We were absolutely gutted. We had a review with our consultant, who said there was no explanation for the three failed embryo transfers. He encouraged us to continue with the third and final funded round when we were ready to do so.

It took a little bit of time to find the courage to continue, but we went ahead with our third egg collection in February 2023 and managed to get four genetically normal embryos (which is great news)! I have just started taking my FET cycle medication and, despite it not being an easy road, we still hold onto hope.

> *Before we began IVF, I hadn't heard of anyone else who has had PGT and didn't know much about the process. I hope my story will educate others a little about genetic abnormalities affecting fertility (such as translocations) and PGT. I also want people to know that, despite it not being smooth, we can find the courage to keep going. There is always hope.*

3. **Preimplantation Genetic Testing for Monogenic Conditions (PGT-M)** screens embryos for single-gene (monogenic) conditions, so it is designed for couples or individuals who are at risk of passing on a known genetic condition caused by a mutation in a specific gene rather than a large piece of a chromosome. These genetic abnormalities are much smaller than those detected by PGT-A and PGT-SR, so the technologies needed to perform PGT-M are different. PGT-M often requires a longer set up time prior to IVF, as well as DNA samples from the egg provider, sperm provider, and their parents. PGT-M identifies which embryos are at risk of being affected by or carriers of the disease in question, and which are at a low risk of developing the condition (see section on genetic carrier screening in Chapter 5 for more information).

Amy's Story

Our fertility journey did not begin well. After an unexplained stillbirth at thirty-seven weeks and a termination of pregnancy for medical reasons (TFMR), we discovered that I am a carrier of a rare genetic disorder. If we didn't do genetic carrier screening, I may have never known that I was a carrier of this genetic condition that could be passed on to my child. This realization helped us move forward because we learned that we could do IVF with PGT-M (monogenic) to test our embryos for the same genetic disorder.

After completing an IVF cycle with PGT-M, we ended up with three healthy embryos that are not affected by the genetic disorder and are confidently moving forward toward our next steps.

I hope that my story helps others embarking on their fertility journeys feel less alone and gives them strength to not give up.

PGT-A Results

PGT-A results fall into several categories, each with distinct implications for embryo viability and transfer decisions:

- **Euploid:** This is a normal result which indicates that no chromosomal abnormalities are present in the cells in a biopsy sample. Embryos with this type of result usually have the highest chance of implantation and ongoing pregnancy, though an embryo's morphology influences its success, as well. A euploid result cannot guarantee implantation, live birth, or a healthy baby due to testing limitations.
- **Aneuploid:** This is an abnormal result and means that a chromosomal abnormality was detected in the biopsied cells. The meaning of the result depends on what type of chromosomal abnormality was detected. Different types of aneuploid results include:
  - **Whole chromosome aneuploid:** an entire copy of a chromosome is missing and/or present. Types of whole chromosome aneuploidy include:
    - **Monosomy**: there is one copy of a chromosome instead of two. This can be represented on a report by a minus sign followed by the missing chromosome number (e.g., −22 for monosomy 22).
    - **Trisomy**: there are three copies of a chromosome instead of two. This can be represented on a report by a plus sign followed by the extra chromosome number (e.g., +16 for trisomy 16).

    Studies show that this type of result is highly accurate. When whole chromosome aneuploidy is detected on PGT-A, it is usually present throughout the entire blastocyst, including the inner cell mass (the cells that can develop into the fetus). The incidence of these types of chromosome errors increase as the age of the egg provider increases.[1]
  - **Segmental aneuploid:** a piece or segment of a chromosome is missing or extra, rather than the entire copy. Segmental aneuploidies are often called deletions (partial monosomy) and duplications (partial trisomy):
    - A deletion is when part of a chromosome is missing. On a report, "del" or a minus sign may be used to indicate a segmental deletion.
    - A duplication is when part of a chromosome is extra. On a report "dup" or a plus sign may be used to indicate a segmental duplication.

The letters "p" or "q" are often included in this type of result to indicate whether the deleted or duplicated segment impacted the p or q arm of the chromosome. For example, del(13)(q22-qter) would indicate a deletion on chromosome 13 spanning from band 22 on the q arm to the terminus (end) of the q arm.

Studies show that this type of result is less accurate than whole chromosome aneuploidy. Embryos with this type of result are more likely to be mosaic.[2] This type of aneuploidy does not happen more frequently with increasing parental age.[3,4,5] Finally, not all PGT-A laboratories are able to detect or report this type of result, and the size of the segments that can be detected (the detection threshold) varies between labs.

- **Complex aneuploid:** This is defined as a result with at least three chromosome abnormalities. The interpretation of the result depends on the specific abnormalities that are detected. Note that this term is not used by all laboratories, and the definition can vary depending on the PGT-A lab.
- **Chaotic:** This is defined as a result with six or more chromosome abnormalities. The interpretation of the result depends on the individual abnormalities that are detected. Note that this term is not used by all laboratories, and the definition can vary depending on the PGT-A lab. This type of result may also have a lower chance of accurately reflecting the genetics of the entire embryo.[6] More research is needed, as studies on this result type are small and limited to a single PGT-A laboratory. It is unknown if research about this result type is applicable to all PGT-A laboratories.

• **Mosaic:** This intermediate result indicates that some of the tested cells contained normal chromosomes (euploid) and other tested cells contained abnormal chromosomes (aneuploid). Mosaic results are often described as a low-level or high-level based on the proportion of abnormal cells in the biopsied sample. Embryos with mosaic results may have lower implantation rates and higher miscarriage rates compared to embryos with euploid results, however, many studies are starting to show that low-level mosaic embryos may have outcomes similar to euploid embryos.[7,8,9] Babies born from mosaic embryos do not appear to have increased risks of chromosomal abnormalities or birth defects compared to euploid embryos.[10,11,12] Not all PGT-A laboratories can detect or report mosaicism. Additionally, some labs allow individual clinics and doctors to opt in or out of mosaic reporting.

- **No result:** This result means that the PGT-A lab was not able to provide a result for this embryo. This can be because there was no DNA or not enough DNA obtained from the biopsied cells, because the DNA obtained was of poor quality, or because the data obtained from the test did not clearly show a result. Embryos with this result type often have the same chance of being euploid as untested embryos.[13] The likelihood of euploidy is primarily based on the age of the egg provider.

PGT Results and Embryo Transfer Status

Each IVF clinic or physician may have their own policies or preferences regarding which embryos they consider suitable for transfer based on PGT results. Clinics that offer PGT-A often transfer euploid embryos before considering embryos with other types of results for transfer. For clinics with strict policies, only euploid embryos are considered suitable for transfer. Many clinics allow embryos with no result or mosaic results for transfer. Some clinics may only transfer low-level mosaic embryos while others transfer both low- and high-level mosaic embryos. Most clinics do not transfer aneuploid embryos. As our understanding of different types of aneuploid results changes, some clinics may consider specific aneuploid results for transfer, though this is rare.

Determining Normal Versus Abnormal with PGT-A

Most PGT-A performed in 2025 uses Next Generation Sequencing (NGS). This highly-sensitive technology generates multiple data points for each of the twenty-four chromosome These data points are plotted on a graph to assess whether each chromosome has one, two, or three copies, and they may also assess whether there are segmental imbalances (partial deletions or duplications) on the chromosome. These data points are averaged by complex computer algorithms to produce the final result that is recorded in the PGT-A report.

It is normal for there to be some "noise" in the NGS data points. An ideal normal result would show 0% abnormality, but this is rare. A euploid embryo may have data points that slightly deviate from 0%. To account for this, PGT-A laboratories that use NGS have different ranges or thresholds for what they consider a euploid, aneuploid, and mosaic result. There is currently no universal standardization for these thresholds, so they vary between PGT labs. Here are some common examples of thresholds used to call PGT-A results:

PGT-A Laboratory 1	PGT-A Laboratory 2
Euploid: <20% abnormality	Euploid: <30% abnormality
Low-level mosaic: 20–40% abnormality	Low-level mosaic: 30–50% abnormality
High-level mosaic: >40–80% abnormality	High-level mosaic: >50–70% abnormality
Aneuploid: >80% abnormality	Aneuploid: >70% abnormality

For lab 1, the data points can deviate away from normal by up to 20 percent and the test would still show a euploid result.

Let's keep using lab 1 as an example. You can think of the NGS data graph like a thermometer, where the goal is for the temperature to be at zero degrees. This would be a euploid (normal) result. It's normal for there to be some noise in the NGS data, just like it is normal for temperature to fluctuate a bit. As long as the temperature doesn't rise or drop by more than 20 degrees, this is considered normal. If the temperature rises or drops by 80 degrees, this is significant and is considered clearly abnormal. If the temperature rises or drops by 20–80 degrees, this isn't normal, but it isn't considered abnormal either, and we consider this an intermediate or a mosaic result.

Mosaic Embryos

It's important to understand that a mosaic result on PGT-A does not necessarily mean that the embryo itself is mosaic. A mosaic embryo is an embryo that we know is made of some euploid and some aneuploid cells. There can be a few possible reasons for a mosaic result obtained from PGT-A:

- The embryo is a true mosaic, and both euploid and aneuploid cells were included in the biopsy.
- The result is a false positive and doesn't truly represent the genetic status of the embryo. False positives can occur due to sample contamination, or due to processes that occur during testing that make it look like the embryo is mosaic when it is actually euploid or fully aneuploid.[14]

True mosaicism typically results from an error in mitosis (cell division), the biological process the process by which cells divide and replicate. Once the egg and sperm cell have come together to produce a fertilized egg (zygote), mitosis is the process the fertilized egg will use to grow and become a blastocyst.

Each of our cells normally has forty-six chromosomes (23 pairs) in total. When mitosis occurs, the chromosomes replicate themselves so that there are ninety-two in total. The cell then divides, and the ninety-two chromosomes divide with it. The result should be two cells, each with identical copies of the original forty-six chromosomes.

Errors can occur when cells undergo mitosis. If the ninety-two chromosomes do not split evenly among the two new cells that form, it can cause the two new cells to have the incorrect number of chromosomes. One cell may receive an extra chromosome (trisomy) and one cell may be missing the same chromosome (monosomy). These cells have chromosomal abnormalities and would be considered aneuploid. However, the embryo still has the euploid cells that it started with, but now it also has new aneuploid cells. Since the embryo now has both euploid and aneuploid cells, it is considered a mosaic embryo.

This is just one way that mosaicism can occur. Other, rarer mechanisms can lead to mosaicism, as well.

Reasons to Perform PGT-A

There are many reasons why someone may want to consider PGT-A as part of their IVF treatment.

- PGT-A screens for common chromosomal disorders such as Down syndrome or Patau syndrome. The frequency of these disorders increases as the age of the egg provider increases. For some, having the ability to screen for these disorders before an embryo is transferred into the uterus is a benefit of PGT-A.

- PGT-A can be used as a tool to help prioritize embryos for transfer. Without PGT-A, embryos are often prioritized based on morphology (how they look under the microscope). However, embryos with good morphology do not necessarily have normal chromosomes.[15,16] Knowing which embryos show euploid results can help prioritize those embryos for transfer, potentially speeding up the time to an ongoing pregnancy by avoiding transfer of embryos with aneuploid chromosomes that are likely to fail to implant or miscarry.

- If someone has had multiple embryo transfers that have failed to implant or lead to miscarriage, they may wish to undergo PGT-A to have a better understanding of why their embryo transfers have been unsuccessful. Fertility specialists may assume that aneuploidy is the reason why transfers are failing when PGT-A is not used. Transferring embryos with euploid results helps doctors rule aneuploidy out as a potential cause of transfer failure and work to better understand the factors at play.
- In some countries, including the United States, you can learn the sex of an embryo via PGT-A. For some individuals this information is valuable either for informational purposes, family balancing, or to reduce the risk of a genetic disease that is sex-linked (affects one sex more commonly or exclusively).
- Without the use of PGT-A, it is more common to transfer more than one embryo in order to improve success rates. This is because we expect that some of the embryos transferred will be aneuploid and will not lead to an ongoing pregnancy. However, when multiple embryos are transferred, it is possible that more than one will implant and lead to an ongoing twin pregnancy or a pregnancy with higher order multiples (triplets, quadruplets, etc.). These pregnancies can cause complications that can put the health of the babies and the person carrying the pregnancy at risk. Transfer of a single embryo with a euploid result allows for high pregnancy rates without the increased risk of multiple pregnancies.

PGT-A Accuracy

Accuracy in PGT-A depends on the genetic testing lab and their individual testing technologies and procedures. Accuracy can also mean a few different things when it comes to PGT-A:

1. Did the test correctly identify the chromosomal status of the cells that it tested?

    Most laboratories will perform studies to answer this question about their test and will include information about this type of accuracy on their report.

2. Do the biopsied cells accurately represent the genetics of the entire embryo, including the rest of the trophectoderm and the inner cell mass?

Laboratories may not answer this question for their test specifically. This is harder to confirm and typically assessed through research studies rather than individual lab reports. Accuracy varies depending on the type of result. We'll discuss this further in the section "Should I have an embryo tested again?".

3. Do embryos with aneuploid results fail to result in ongoing pregnancies and live births, as expected?

    This is the least studied aspect of PGT-A accuracy due to ethical concerns. The answer to this likely depends on the subtype of aneuploidy. You can discuss the chance that an embryo with an aneuploid result will lead to an ongoing pregnancy with your doctor or genetic counselor.

Embryo Re-Biopsy

Re-testing an embryo after receiving a PGT-A result involves thawing the embryo, performing a second trophectoderm biopsy, and re-freezing the embryo while awaiting the new result. Though there is an increased risk of embryo damage during these processes, limited data suggest that over 90 percent of good-quality embryos survive and remain suitable for transfer. Whether re-biopsy is appropriate depends on the embryo's appearance, your clinic's policies, and your healthcare team's assessment. The usefulness of re-biopsy varies based on the initial PGT-A result:

- **No result.** Re-biopsy may be helpful when the initial test was inconclusive or yielded no result.
- **Whole chromosome aneuploidy.** Re-biopsy is usually not recommended for an embryo that shows an aneuploid result that affects a whole chromosome (monosomy or trisomy). Studies show that this type of result usually affects all cells of the embryo, including cells that were not tested. Repeat testing often confirms the original result.[17,18]
- **Mosaic.** Re-biopsy of an embryo with a mosaic PGT-A result is also not recommended because, no matter what result we see in the second test, it will not contradict the initial mosaic result. A mosaic result suggests that

some cells of the embryo are euploid and some cells of the embryo are aneuploid. Therefore, if we re-test and get a euploid result from the new sample, this is still consistent with the embryo being mosaic since we know mosaic embryos contain euploid cells. The same concept applies if we receive an aneuploid result with the new sample. We know mosaic embryos also contain aneuploid cells, so getting an aneuploid result is still consistent with the embryo being mosaic.

- **Segmental aneuploidy.** Research suggests that embryos with segmental aneuploidy results on PGT-A have a higher chance of being mosaic even when the initial biopsy did not show mosaicism. There may also be a higher chance for these results to be false positives, meaning that the abnormality may not be present in the embryo at all.[19] For these reasons, re-biopsy of embryos with this type of result may be helpful in understanding the genetic makeup of the embryo. Girardi et al. (2020) developed a model to predict the chance that an embryo with this type of result will have a euploid inner cell mass. It is based on the size of the segmental aneuploidy detected in the initial biopsy and whether or not the same aneuploidy was detected in the re-biopsy sample. More research is needed. Additionally, a euploid result on rebiopsy may be enough for us to consider the embryo mosaic for the segmental abnormality, but it can be argued that it is not enough for the embryo itself to be considered euploid.

- **Chaotic.** Very small research studies performed by a single PGT-A laboratory suggest that chaotic results may be less accurate at representing the genetics of the entire embryo than other types of aneuploid results. To date, there is a single case report of an embryo with this type of result leading to a healthy live birth. Additionally, when a small number of embryos with chaotic results were re-biopsied, approximately 38 percent showed euploid results. The authors suggest that re-biopsy may be considered after genetic counseling and informed consent.[20] It is unknown whether these findings apply to embryos with chaotic results at other PGT-A laboratories.

Age and Aneuploidy

Women are born with all of the eggs they will ever have, but these eggs are immature at birth. These eggs begin with two sets of chromosomes. Around the time of ovulation and fertilization, the eggs undergo processes that cause them to go from having two sets of chromosomes to one. As immature eggs age, this process occurs with more errors increasing the risk of aneuploidy. With this in mind, PGT-A is sometimes considered more frequently for women who are considered to be of advanced reproductive age. The rate of aneuploidy in eggs increases slowly each year. The rates of aneuploidy rise after the age of thirty-five, and aneuploidy rates rise more noticeably more quickly after the age of forty.[21]

While age is a factor in deciding whether to pursue PGT-A, it should be considered alongside cost, timing, testing accuracy, number of blastocysts, and personal goals and values.

Sperm and Aneuploidy

Some embryo aneuploidies do originate from the sperm, but at a much lower frequency compared to the egg. It is believed that the majority of whole chromosome aneuploidies (the most common type of aneuploidy) originate from the eggs. Segmental aneuploidies are often mitotic, meaning that they don't originate in the egg or the sperm, but happen due to errors that occur after egg and sperm come together. However, if a segmental aneuploidy is meiotic (originates from the egg or sperm from the beginning), it is more likely to originate from the sperm.[22]

Other PGT-A Considerations

PGT-A is a test that can be useful for many individuals, but it is essential to understand the benefits, risks, and limitations of the testing before proceeding with it.

The differences in how PGT labs perform their tests can lead to dramatic changes in euploidy rates and live birth rates between the labs.[23]

Often, laboratories design their test and begin offering it to patients without extensive research into the accuracy or limitations of the test. This means that our understanding of the results can change over time, sometimes after you have made the decision to discard an embryo. Certified Genetic Counselors who specialize in fertility genetics are best positioned to provide education about the benefits and limitations of PGT-A, as well as help you understand the results that you receive from the testing. You can find a genetic counselor on the National Society of Genetic Counselors website https://findageneticcounselor.nsgc.org or by asking your fertility clinic for more information.

Conclusions

PGT has become a common practice in IVF cycles. There are various types of PGT and implications for their use. Understanding your PGT results can help determine how to proceed with your treatment.

Chapter 9
Failed Implantation and Pregnancy Loss

The information in this chapter was contributed by Geoffrey Sher, co-founder and associate medical director of Sher Fertility Solutions (SFS).

A pregnancy begins once an embryo successfully implants into the endometrium (uterine lining). As discussed in Chapter 3, the endometrium must be thickened and ready to receive an embryo prior to implantation. Once the embryo enters the uterus, there is a small window of time during which embryo implantation is possible. During this window, the embryo and endometrium engage in "crosstalk," which allows the following events to unfold:

- **Apposition**: the embryo finds a suitable location for implantation and adheres to the endometrium
- **Implantation**: the embryo begins to burrow into the endometrium
- **Invasion**: the embryo penetrates the endometrial epithelium (layer of cells) and establishes blood vessels that connect it to the maternal (or gestational carrier's) blood supply. This blood supply provides oxygen and nutrients that are essential for development throughout the pregnancy.

Central to the success of reproduction is the "seed and soil" analogy: a healthy, competent "seed" (embryo) must be planted into receptive "soil" (endometrium). Failure to meet these conditions can result in failed implantation or pregnancy loss.

Reproductive failure refers to the inability to reproduce and encompasses both infertility (the inability to conceive a pregnancy) and recurrent pregnancy loss (the inability to maintain a pregnancy). In approximately 75 percent of cases, reproductive failure is due to embryo incompetence, most often caused by chromosomal abnormalities (aneuploidy) in the embryo's cells. In the remaining 25 percent of cases, reproductive failure is linked to structural abnormalities of the uterus and/or immunologic implantation dysfunction (IID).

Chapters 2 and 3 explore common causes of male and female infertility. This chapter will focus on causes of reproductive failure *after* an embryo is transferred into a uterus.

Pregnancy Loss

Though no one wants to hear it, it's important to understand that pregnancy loss can occur at any stage and almost always causes feelings of sadness, grief, and anger. Chapter 10 explores these emotions and offers options for support.

An early pregnancy loss (EPL, also known as miscarriage or spontaneous abortion) typically occurs within the first trimester, though variations in the definition exist. EPLs account for roughly 80 percent of all pregnancy losses.

The most common cause of *sporadic* (not recurrent) EPL is embryo incompetence (the inability to successfully implant and develop into a live birth), which is typically due to aneuploidy (chromosomal abnormalities, see Chapter 8). Conversely, *recurrent* EPL is more often linked to implantation dysfunction (errors during implantation).

Types of EPLs include a(n):

- **Chemical (biochemical) pregnancy**: a pregnancy is confirmed by elevated hCG hormone levels in the blood or urine, but lost before an ultrasound can visualize the pregnancy.

- **Missed (silent) miscarriage**: the embryo or fetus stops developing, but the body does not expel the tissue from the uterus. There are often no signs of miscarriage because pregnancy symptoms may persist due to continued hormone production.

- **Anembryonic pregnancy (blighted ovum)**: the embryo implants into the endometrium and a gestational sac forms, but fetal cells are nonviable. These can sometimes cause missed miscarriages since pregnancy hormone levels can continue to rise and cause pregnancy symptoms to persist. Anembryonic pregnancies are the cause of roughly 50 percent of first-trimester losses.

- **Molar pregnancy (hydatidiform mole)**: abnormal fertilization leads to rapid placental cell growth, but the fetal cells are nonviable. The placental cells grow and can form a benign tumor inside of the uterus that can become cancerous if left untreated. There are two types of molar pregnancies:
  - **Complete**: an egg with no chromosomes is fertilized by one or two sperm. In other words, the embryo only contains DNA from the sperm, making it nonviable.
  - **Partial**: an egg is fertilized by two sperm (or one sperm with two sets of DNA), resulting in an embryo with an extra set of DNA. The placenta develops abnormally and, while the embryo/fetus may initially begin to develop, it is often severely malformed due to the chromosomal abnormalities and cannot survive.
- **Ectopic pregnancy**: while this isn't a natural pregnancy loss, it is still an EPL. Ectopic pregnancies are life-threatening conditions in which implantation occurs outside the uterus, typically in the fallopian tube (a tubal pregnancy). Unfortunately, ectopic pregnancies must be terminated to prevent severe complications, including rupture, hemorrhage, and death.

Late pregnancy loss (LPL) occurs after the first trimester and is often caused by:

- Anatomical abnormalities of the uterus and/or cervix. In particular, cervical incompetence (weakness of the neck of the cervix which causes it to dilate prematurely under the pressure of the growing pregnancy) is one of the most common causes of LPL.
- Developmental (congenital) abnormalities (structural defects in the uterus that are present from birth)
- Uterine fibroids
- Intrauterine growth restriction (IUGR)
- Placental abruption (the placenta detaches from the inner wall of the uterus before delivery, either partially or completely.)
- Premature rupture of the membranes (PROM) or Preterm Prelabor Rupture of Membranes (PPROM) (the amniotic sac is broken prematurely)
- Very premature labor

Note: Stillbirth (intrauterine fetal demise) refers to the loss of a fetus after twenty weeks of gestation.

> ### *Maya's Story*
>
> *We had the privilege to go through IVF, so we got to know our daughter Maya from when she was no more than a little embryo. And we were in love. And we were heavily monitored. We went through genetic screening, genetic testing and ICSI, three early ultrasounds and lots of blood work. And Maya was thriving. We graduated from our fertility clinic, transferred our care to our OB (obstetrician), and had another ultrasound.*
>
> *Maya was perfect. At fourteen weeks, we had another ultrasound—because why not see her again?—and she was beautiful. We started her nursery, we started to tell people, we took a breath and let our guard down.*
>
> *But then my wife started bleeding on the way to her sixteen-week check up. Our OB checked for a heart beat, which was 144, and she did another ultrasound. Maya was perfect. My wife was sent home awaiting a diagnostic ultrasound in the morning, with the advice to try to breathe because our daughter was fine. Maya was fine.*
>
> *And she died anyway. The experts in the room did not expect this outcome, and she died anyway. We had a team of incredible doctors and genuine human beings. And Maya died anyway.*
>
> *This is the limit of modern medicine. IVF has come a long way, but there is still so much we don't know. With that said, we will forever fight to push the limits of modern medicine and IVF forward. We are on a mission to change the odds for other families in honor of our Maya.*
>
> *Maya grew wings before we were ready, but her grace will fly high, her strength will soar, and with our help, she will change the world. We began the Maya's Wings Foundation to help improve health outcomes of IVF-related pregnancies and eliminate preventable pregnancy loss for ALL.*

Recurrent pregnancy loss (RPL) refers to multiple clinical pregnancy losses, though definitions may vary between clinics and research studies. Significant progress has been made in understanding the mechanisms involved in RPL, and these mechanisms can be broken down into two categories:

1. Genetic and/or structural chromosomal abnormalities in the embryo such as aneuploidy (abnormal number of chromosomes) and unbalanced translocations (segments of chromosomes are rearranged in a way that disrupts genetic balance). These abnormalities often result in embryos that are unable to implant or develop into a live birth.

2. Problems involving the uterine environment that impair embryo implantation and development. These include:

   - Inadequate thickening of the uterine lining, typically from deficient blood flow to the uterine lining or abnormal hormone production.
   - Structural irregularities in the uterine cavity, such as polyps, fibroids, intrauterine adhesions, or congenital anomalies (e.g., uterine septum).
   - Hormonal imbalances (e.g., progesterone deficiency or luteal phase defects). These often result in missed ("hidden" or occult) RPL, where losses occur before clinical detection.
   - Immunologic implantation dysfunction (IID), including thyroid disorders and diabetes mellitus.
   - Thrombophilia, which can interfere with blood supply to the developing embryo (see below).
   - Chronic inflammation of the uterine lining (endometritis).

When individuals or couples experience RPL, a thorough clinical workup is often recommended to identify potential underlying causes. This workup might include a(n):

- Mid-cycle pelvic ultrasound to assess the thickness and configuration of the uterine lining.
- Sonohysterogram (SHG, or saline infusion sonogram) or hysteroscopy to evaluate the uterine cavity for structural abnormalities.
- Alloimmune (both partners) and autoimmune (female partner) evaluation.
- Hormonal assessment of ovarian, pituitary, thyroid, and kidney function.
- Chromosomal analysis (karyotype) of both partners to detect translocations (one piece of a chromosome breaks off and attaches to a different chromosome) or other chromosomal abnormalities.

Causes of Reproductive Failure

Embryo Incompetence

Embryo incompetence refers to an embryo's inability to successfully implant, develop normally, and result in a healthy live birth. There are multiple causes of embryo incompetence, including poor embryo quality, intrinsic abnormalities, and aneuploidy.

Poor embryo quality. An embryo's quality reflects its potential to implant and develop into a healthy pregnancy. In IVF, embryo quality is evaluated based on an embryo's unique appearance (morphology) and rate of development. An embryo is considered "high-quality" if its appearance and rate of development fall within expected ranges (see Chapter 7). Embryos that are abnormal in appearance or delayed in development are labeled poor-quality embryos.

An embryo's quality can affect its competence. In general, the lower the quality of an embryo, the lower its chance of implanting into the uterine lining and resulting in a live birth. Additionally, poor-quality embryos are less likely to be euploid (have the correct number of chromosomes) than high-quality embryos.

It's important to note that, despite their lower success rates, poor-quality embryos can result in healthy live births.

Intrinsic abnormalities. Some embryos have internal issues that affect their ability to implant or develop, including:

- Impaired mitochondrial function, which limits the embryo's energy production
- Abnormal gene expression, which disrupts key developmental processes

Unfortunately, there is currently no way to reliably visualize or screen embryos for intrinsic abnormalities.

Aneuploidy. Sporadic pregnancy loss is most often due to embryo aneuploidy (the embryo's cells have chromosome abnormalities, see Chapter 8). Aneuploid embryos are at an increased risk of failed implantation and miscarriage. Unfortunately, the incidence of embryo aneuploidy increases with age, though it can occur at any time. Many individuals who undergo IVF choose to have their embryos undergo preimplantation genetic testing for aneuploidy (PGT-A) to identify which of their embryos have the correct number of chromosomes (i.e., are euploid) before they are transferred into the uterus.

While any embryo can technically be transferred, high-quality embryos (especially those which are deemed euploid via PGT-A) are normally transferred first to optimize the chances of implantation and live birth.

Uterine Lesions

Uterine lesions are abnormalities or growths within or on the uterus that can interfere with embryo implantation and development. Depending on their type, size, and location, lesions may:

- Distort the shape of the uterine cavity

- Reduce blood flow to the endometrium, which can deprive the embryo/fetus of the oxygen and nutrients required for survival and development
- Physically block an embryo from reaching or attaching to an implantation site
- Trigger a local inflammatory response
- Block the fallopian tubes, which interferes with sperm transport to the egg and embryo transport to the uterus
- Cause abnormal uterine contractions
- Alter endometrial receptivity to an embryo

Even small uterine lesions can negatively impact implantation, so many clinics perform diagnostic tests such as a hysterosalpingo-contrast sonography (HyCoSy), hysterosalpingography (HSG), sonohysterogram (SHG), or hysteroscopy prior to an embryo transfer to identify and treat uterine lesions as needed. Common endometrial lesions include:

- Endometrial polyps are overgrowths of endometrial tissue that protrude into the uterine cavity. They can vary in size and location. While not all polyps interfere with implantation and require removal, they can be surgically removed via a procedure known as a polypectomy to optimize pregnancy outcomes.
- Uterine fibroids (leiomyomas) are noncancerous growths (tumors) that are derived from the muscular (middle) layer of the uterus. There are various types of fibroids, and they can develop throughout the uterus and vary in size. Submucosal fibroids, which are located just beneath the endometrium and can protrude into the uterine cavity, are most likely to affect infertility. It's possible to have multiple fibroids at one time.
- Adenomyosis is a condition in which endometrial-like tissue grows into the middle, muscular layer of the uterus.
- Asherman's syndrome refers to the presence of scar tissue (adhesions) on the endometrium, typically a result of inflammation following:
    - An incomplete miscarriage
    - Pelvic inflammatory disease (PID)
    - Chronic endometritis
    - Uterine surgery (e.g.,dilation and curettage (D&C), dilation and evacuation (D&E), C-section, or uterine ablation)

Müllerian (Congenital) Uterine Anomalies

The uterus, fallopian tubes, cervix, and the upper two-thirds of the vagina are formed during early fetal development from structures known as the Müllerian ducts. Errors in this development may result in congenital anomalies that can interfere with implantation and pregnancy outcomes, though some congenital abnormalities do not impact pregnancies. Some congenital abnormalities can be treated surgically, but others unfortunately cannot. Common Müllerian anomalies include:

- **Müllerian agenesis (MRKH syndrome)**: partial or complete absence of uterus, cervix, and/or vagina
- **Cervical agenesis**: some or all of the cervix does not develop
- **Unicornuate uterus**: only one half of the uterus forms
- **Uterus didelphys**: two separate uteri and cervices (and sometimes vaginas) form instead of one
- **Bicornuate uterus**: the uterus is heart-shaped with a deep indentation at the top (fundus)
- **Septate uterus**: the uterine cavity is completely or partially separated by a septum (wall of tissue)

Thin Endometrium

Prior to embryo implantation, the endometrium (uterine lining) thickens with blood and tissues that support embryo implantation and development in response to rising estradiol (E2) and progesterone (P4) levels from the ovaries. In some circumstances, the endometrium is unable to respond to E2 and P4, and therefore does not thicken enough to support successful embryo implantation and development. The main causes of a thin endometrium are:

- Damage to the endometrium due to:
  - Chronic inflammation (endometritis), often resulting from an incomplete abortion, a miscarriage, a sexually transmitted infection (STI) such as chlamydia or gonorrhea, or childbirth
  - Surgical trauma (e.g., D&C) which can result in the formation of scar tissue (Asherman's syndrome)

- Insensitivity of the endometrium to E2 and/or P4
- Low E2 and/or P4 levels
- Reduced blood flow to the endometrium caused by:
  - Uterine fibroids, especially if they are located beneath the endometrium (submucosal)
  - Adenomyosis
  - Scar tissue
  - Smoking or chronic stress

Treatment of a thin endometrium depends on the cause and should be discussed with a fertility specialist.

Medical Conditions and Medications

Some medical conditions can increase the risk of infertility and pregnancy loss, especially if they are uncontrolled. It is best to manage these conditions before you try to conceive to optimize your chances of success. Common examples include:

- High blood pressure
- Cervical insufficiency (incompetent cervix)
- Endocrine disorders (e.g., PCOS, diabetes, thyroid dysfunction)
- Luteal phase defect (the ovaries do not produce enough progesterone)
- Infections (e.g., Rubella, CMV)
- Obesity
- Malnutrition
- Sexually transmitted infections (STIs) like Chlamydia and Gonorrhea, which which can cause pelvic inflammatory disease (PID)

Foodborne illnesses (e.g., Salmonella, Listeriosis, and Toxoplasmosis) during pregnancy can also increase the risk of pregnancy loss. These are often linked to unpasteurized cheese, raw eggs, or undercooked meat.

Some medications can increase the risk of pregnancy loss. These include Misoprostol, Methotrexate, Retinoids, and NSAIDs. *It is imperative that you consult with your fertility specialist or OBGYN before taking any medications or supplements if you are pregnant or trying to conceive!*

Lifestyle Factors and Environmental Hazards

Certain lifestyle choices and environmental exposures have been shown to increase the incidence of reproductive failure. These factors should especially be avoided before and during pregnancy:

- Smoking and exposure to secondhand smoke, including marijuana and vapes
- Excessive alcohol intake
- The use of illegal substances
- High doses of caffeine

Other environmental hazards that can affect a pregnancy include exposure to:

- Heavy metals (e.g., lead, mercury, arsenic)
- Toxic chemicals (e.g., paint thinners, pesticides)
- Radiation
- Air pollution

Immunologic Implantation Dysfunction (IID)

For pregnancy to occur, the immune system must accept the embryo. Normally, the body's immune system attacks foreign substances (bacteria, viruses, foreign tissue grafts/transplantation). So, how is an embryo, which contains genetic material from another individual (the sperm source), often able to safely implant into the uterine lining and thrive without being rejected? The answer lies in the unique and complex immunologic adaptations that occur during implantation. These changes allow the maternal (or gestational carrier's) immune system to recognize the embryo as safe, rather than as a foreign invader. In essence, the immune system is reprogrammed to tolerate the embryo, enabling it to implant and develop rather than be attacked.

Immunological implantation dysfunction (IID) refers to a condition where the mother's (or gestational carrier's) immune system fails to properly adapt, resulting in interference with embryo implantation. It is considered a significant cause of infertility and recurrent pregnancy loss.

The following conditions may raise a suspicion of IID:

1. A diagnosis of endometriosis or suspected endometriosis (heavy/painful menstruation, pain with ovulation or deep penetration).
2. A personal or family history of autoimmune hypothyroidism or hyperthyroidism, which is often associated with elevated TSH levels.
3. Elevated blood levels of antithyroid or anti-TSH antibodies.
4. Family or personal history of any disease believed to have an autoimmune cause (e.g.,Lupus erythematosus, rheumatoid arthritis, dermatomyositis, scleroderma).
5. Presence of antiphospholipid antibodies.
6. Unexplained infertility.
7. Unexplained IVF failure.
8. Recurrent implantation failure.
9. Recurrent pregnancy loss.
10. A history of miscarrying a genetically normal fetus.
11. Secondary infertility (inability to conceive after a previous successful pregnancy).
12. Unexplained intrauterine growth restriction, particularly in late pregnancy loss involving a genetically normal baby.

What Normally Occurs During Implantation

Implantation and early pregnancy depend on a carefully orchestrated immunological dialogue between the embryo's trophoblast cells (which form the outer layer of the embryo and directly interact with the endometrium, or uterine lining) and the maternal (or carrier's) immune system. When an embryo begins implanting into the endometrium (which later becomes known as the decidua), a few events normally occur:

1. Several genes (called HLA genes) on the embryo's trophoblast cells turn on (activate).

2. This activation regulates the activity of two types of immune cells that are present in the endometrium: uterine natural killer (NK) cells and cytotoxic T cells.
3. NK and T cells release *very specific* amounts of proteins known as cytokines that aid in embryo implantation. There are three varieties of cytokines, two of which play defining roles in implantation:
    1. TH-1 cytokines promote controlled destruction of trophoblast cells (to prevent the embryo from implanting too far into the uterus) and also cause blood to clot.
    2. TH-2 cytokines encourage growth and expansion of the trophoblast into the endometrium vascular (blood vessel) development, and placental formation.

The balance between TH1 and TH-2 cytokines is crucial for optimal implantation and placental development.

Errors in Natural Killer Cell Activation (NKa) Affect Implantation

Embryo implantation may be compromised when natural killer (NK) cells (and to a lesser extent, cytotoxic T cells) release an excessive and disproportionate amount of TH-1 cytokines that attack the trophoblast cells of the embryo. This can damage the trophoblast cells and prevent them from proliferating, differentiating, and properly implanting into the uterine lining. This can cause implantation dysfunction and pregnancy loss because the trophoblast cells (which develop into the placenta) do not establish a strong connection to the maternal (or carrier's) blood supply. Further, excessive TH-1 cytokine release can trigger excessive blood clotting and inflammation where the embryo is implanting, which can be hostile to the developing embryo.

Types of IID and NK Cell Activation

There are two types of IID:
    1. **Alloimmune implantation dysfunction.** Most human cells have twenty-three pairs of chromosomes-one set from the sperm and one set from the egg that created us-in each of our cells. These chromosomes contain many genes (segments of DNA) that provide instructions for building and maintaining our bodies. While all humans have the same set of genes, the specific DNA

sequences within each gene can vary slightly from person to person. These are known as variants (alleles), or variations of the same gene.

Let's use an analogy to understand this better. You see hundreds of dogs in a park. They are all dogs (the same gene), but they differ in their fur colors and sizes. One is large with brown fur. Another is small with black and tan fur. These are variants.

What's interesting to think of is that, in each of our cells, we have two sets of chromosomes that both contain the same genes (e.g., the genes for eye or hair color), but that doesn't mean that the genes on both sets of chromosomes have the same variants. For example, you might have the variants for blue eyes on the set of chromosomes you inherited from your mother, and the variants for brown eyes on the set of chromosomes that you inherited from your father. Same gene (eye color), different variants of that gene.

So, where are we going with all of this?

There is a specific gene, called the DQ Alpha gene, on everyone's sixth chromosomes. DQ Alpha genes are part of the human leukocyte antigen (HLA) system, which helps the immune system recognize what's "self" and what's "non-self." Like all genes, there are many variants of the DQ Alpha gene.

Note: for simplicity, we will use the example of a male and female naturally conceiving a pregnancy.

Though the DQ Alpha variant itself doesn't harm an embryo, it can become an issue if the male and female have the *exact* same DQ Alpha variant on one or both of their sixth chromosomes. This is rare since so many DQ Alpha variants exist, but this could cause some or all of the male's sperm cells to have the exact same DQ Alpha variant as the cells in the female's body.

Let's call this variant "Variant 1." The female's cells contain Variant 1, and so do some (if the male has one set of chromosomes with Variant 1) or all (if both of the male's sixth chromosomes contain Variant 1) of his sperm cells. If one of his sperm cells that contain Variant 1 fertilizes the female's egg, the embryo's chromosomes will also contain Variant 1 (inherited from the sperm). So, now the female's cells have Variant 1 and so does the embryo inside of her uterus. Surprisingly, her body will likely attack this embryo.

This is because the uterine immune system is programmed to only accept embryos with *different* DQ Alpha gene variants than its own. This is known as "alloimmune recognition." When the DQ Alpha variants are identical, the uterine immune system gets confused because the embryo is "too similar" to it. The immune system responds by releasing natural killer (NK) cells that attack the embryo. Usually, this will lead to reproductive failure.

In cases of paternal-maternal DQ Alpha matching, it will often take several pregnancies for NK cell activation to build to the point that women will present with clinical evidence of alloimmune implantation dysfunction. Sometimes, it starts off with one or two live births, whereupon NK/T cell activity starts to build, leading to one or more early miscarriages. Eventually, the NK/T cell activation is so high that subsequent pregnancies can be lost before the individual is even aware that she was pregnant. At this point, she is often diagnosed with secondary, "unexplained" infertility.

Alloimmune implantation dysfunction is diagnosed by testing the blood of both the male and female partners for matching DQ Alpha genes and assessing NK/T cell activation in the female partner's blood.

There are two types of DQ Alpha/HLA genetic matching:

- **Partial DQ Alpha genetic matching**: When only one of the male's DQ Alpha variants matches one of the female's, only half of his sperm cells will contain the same variant as the female (because sperm cells only contain one set of chromosomes) Thus, there is a 50 percent chance that any given embryo created will contain the same matching variant (from the sperm) as the female's DQ Alpha gene. This 50 percent chance is crucial because it implies that not every embryo will trigger the alloimmune response, offering a possibility for a successful pregnancy.

    If NK cell activation is also present, this partial match puts the couple at a significant disadvantage for success. Treatment for partial DQ Alpha match with NK cell activation may differ between clinics but often involves intralipid (IL) infusion and oral prednisone as adjunct therapy. IL infusion may be repeated every two to four weeks after pregnancy is confirmed and continued until the twenty-fourth week of gestation. In these cases, only one embryo should be transferred at a time to minimize the risk of NK cell activation.

- **Total (complete) alloimmune genetic matching**: *Very infrequently,* both of the male's DQ Alpha gene variants match one or both of the female's DQ Alpha gene variant. Here, every sperm and embryo will possess a DQ Alpha gene variant that matches the female's. This scenario, combined with NK cell activation, significantly reduces the chance of a viable pregnancy. In most cases, the use of donor sperm or a gestational carrier (surrogate) with a different DQ Alpha variant may be necessary to "break" the match.

Emily's Story

My husband and I have been trying to conceive since 2017, but we discovered that I have PCOS and endometriosis. After thirteen ovulation inductions we were still not pregnant, so we reluctantly began IVF in early 2022.

We ended up with one frozen embryo from our first cycle and transferred one embryo during our second cycle. Unfortunately, this pregnancy ended in a miscarriage at nine weeks after seeing a low heart rate for four weeks.

After two second opinions and a third IVF cycle that resulted in a chemical pregnancy, we left our clinic because our doctor did not support immune testing. My new doctor performed immune testing, which determined that my husband and I had a complete DQ alpha match. This means that our cells have identical DQ alpha genes, which is rare, and any embryos resulting from my eggs and his sperm have very similar genetic information to my body's cells. In other words, the genetic information in my body's cells and our embryos' cells is too similar. So, when one of our embryos is transferred into my uterus, my body could potentially see the embryo as a threat (because its genetic information is too similar to that of my own cells) and attack the embryo's cells. In particular, my body can release a lot of substances known as cytokines, which can damage the cells that the embryo needs in order to implant.

I did a number of things to improve my egg health before our fourth IVF cycle, including:

- *seeing a naturopath and completing a full gut microbiome testing, which discovered bad bacteria in my gut (which is linked to poor egg health)*
- *Focusing on improving my mental health since I was still in denial after my miscarriage*
- *Taking supplements recommended by our new doctor*
- *Eating better*
- *Not consuming alcohol*
- *Exercising regularly*
- *Completing acupuncture*
- *Changing my stimulation protocol for the first time*

We did our fourth IVF cycle at the new clinic and ended up with five frozen embryos! I believe that all of the changes we made contributed to a better outcome, and I'm going to continue celebrating our victory.

> *Since the last IVF cycle, we have completed our first lymphocyte immunization therapy (LIT) session (this should help regulate my body's immune system so it doesn't attack any transferred embryos) to help combat the DQ Alpha match, and will eventually do our first frozen transfer with a full immune protocol. We are hoping that this is our missing piece.*
>
> *I hope that my story will motivate others to advocate for themselves. I believe that we would have continued to have unsuccessful cycles with our original doctor if we did not advocate for ourselves. We originally felt hopeless, but now we are more hopeful than we've ever been.*

2. **Autoimmune implantation dysfunction.**
The immune system is responsible for protecting us from foreign invaders like viruses and bacteria. However, under certain circumstances, genetic, infectious, toxic, and degenerative influences can result in our *own* body's proteins coming to be regarded as "non-self" ("foreign"). When this happens, the immune system starts to produce antibodies that are directed against our body's *own* proteins. These so-called autoantibodies then start attacking our body's cells/tissues/organs, creating autoimmune diseases such as lupus erythematosus, hypothyroidism, and rheumatoid arthritis.

With autoimmune implantation dysfunction, NK and T cell activation (see above) is already present before the embryo reaches the uterus. Accordingly, in such cases, the pregnancy is usually lost before its presence can be established by a blood pregnancy test or an early ultrasound examination (i.e., it presents as a negative pregnancy test or a biochemical pregnancy).

Those with a personal or family history of autoimmune conditions may experience autoimmune implantation dysfunction, though it can also occur without any known history of autoimmune diseases. Autoimmune implantation dysfunction accounts for more than 75 percent of reproductive failure due to immunologic implantation dysfunction (IID).

The three most common types of autoantibodies involved are antiphospholipid antibodies (APA), antithyroid antibodies (ATA), and possibly, antiovarian antibodies (AOA):

- **Antiphospholipid antibodies (APAs)**. Many women who struggle with IVF failure or recurrent pregnancy loss, as well as those with a personal or family history of autoimmune diseases, often test positive for the presence of antiphospholipid antibodies (APAs). APAs are designed to promote blood clot formation, but certain types of APAs can directly damage an implanting embryo's trophoblast cells and activate NK/T cells.

Sometimes, the body mistakenly produces too many APAs in an autoimmune disorder known as antiphospholipid syndrome (APS). APS is a type of thrombophilia, a condition where the blood has an increased tendency to clot, which can impair the flow of blood between the embryo/fetus and mother (or gestational carrier).

Thrombophilia can cause pregnancy loss (usually after the first trimester) and "unexplained" infertility, and it can be a factor in some cases of "unexplained" IVF failure. Whether (and/or the extent to which) thrombophilia causes first-trimester recurrent pregnancy loss (RPL) is controversial and a subject of ongoing research. Thrombophilia has also been associated with late pregnancy-induced complications such as preeclampsia, premature separation of the placenta (abruptio placentae), placental insufficiency with intrauterine growth restriction, and unexplained intrauterine death. This having been said, most people with thrombophilia experience healthy pregnancies.

Pregnant women with the following predisposing factors should be tested for thrombophilia:

- A personal or family history of thromboembolism (deep vein thrombosis), pulmonary embolism (blood clot in the lung), or cerebrovascular accidents (i.e., strokes)
- A personal history of pregnancy complications such as unexplained intrauterine death, preeclampsia, abruptio placentae, intrauterine growth restriction, and placental insufficiency

Treatment should be initiated as soon as pregnancy is confirmed and continue throughout gestation.

There are also certain reproductive diseases, such as endometriosis, that can increase the production of APAs. More than 50 percent of individuals with endometriosis (regardless of severity) have APAs in their blood, and approximately one third of those who have endometriosis (regardless of severity) show evidence of increased NK cell activity. In these cases, there is an increased likelihood of pregnancy loss.

- **Antithyroid antibodies**.

Up to five percent of women of childbearing age have reduced thyroid hormone activity (hypothyroidism, or Hashimoto's disease). Those with hypothyroidism often manifest with reproductive failure (i.e., infertility, unexplained [often repeated] IVF failure, or recurrent pregnancy loss [RPL]).

In most cases, hypothyroidism is caused by damage to the thyroid gland resulting from autoimmune thyroid disease (AITD). This occurs when the body mistakenly produces autoantibodies that attack the thyroid gland. The increased prevalence of hypothyroidism and AITD in women is likely the result of a combination of genetic factors, estrogen-related effects, and chromosome X abnormalities.

Almost 50 percent of women with AITD do not have activated NK or T cells (see above). This suggests that the autoantibodies themselves may not be a direct cause of reproductive dysfunction. Instead, the activation of NK and T cells, which occurs in about half of the cases with AITD, is likely an accompanying phenomenon that damages the trophoblast cells of the embryo during implantation. Further, thyroid hormones are crucial for embryo development and placental formation, and imbalances caused by AITD can directly affect these processes. Finally, AITD can contribute to a state of chronic low-grade inflammation throughout the body, which can indirectly affect implantation and early placental development.

Treating women who have both antithyroid antibodies along with activated NK and T cells with intralipid (IL) infusions and steroids may improve their chances of successful reproduction. However, women with antithyroid antibodies who do not have activated NK and T cells should not require this treatment.

- **Antiovarian antibodies (autoimmune oophoritis)**

In rare cases, the body's immune system mistakenly produces autoantibodies that attack the ovaries and damage ovarian tissue. This affects ovarian function, which can cause reproductive disorders such as primary ovarian insufficiency (POI), PCOS, and endometriosis. Women with autoimmune diseases are more likely to develop autoimmune oophoritis, though women without autoimmune diseases can also develop it. In cases of autoimmune oophoritis where there is evidence of activated NK cells, treatment will likely be required (as described above).

Treatment Options for IID

Treatment for IID depends on its underlying cause and severity. The goal is to modulate immune activity, particularly natural killer (NK) cell activation and cytokine imbalance, to improve implantation and pregnancy outcomes. Common treatment options might include:

1. Intralipid (IL) therapy, with or without corticosteroids.
2. Intravenous immunoglobulin-G (IVIG) therapy was used in the past to down-regulate activated NK cells. However, concerns about viral transmission and the high cost led to a decline in its use. IVIG can be effective, but IL has become a more favorable and affordable alternative.
3. Corticosteroids (prednisone, dexamethasone) can reduce TH-1 cytokine production by T cells. When combined with IL or IVIG, corticosteroids enhance the implantation process. Treatment typically starts ten to fourteen days before embryo transfer and continues until the tenth week of pregnancy.
4. Low molecular weight heparin (e.g., Clexane, Lovenox) can improve IVF success rates in women with APAs and may also prevent pregnancy loss in certain thrombophilias. It is typically administered subcutaneously once daily from the start of ovarian stimulation.
5. TH-1 Cytokine Blockers (e.g., Enbrel, Humira) may help treat threatened miscarriage caused by T cell/NK cell activation. However, TH-1 cytokines are needed for cellular response during the *early phase of implantation*, so completely blocking them could potentially hinder normal implantation.
6. Lymphocyte Immunization Therapy (LIT) involves injecting the male partner's lymphocytes (a type of white blood cell) into the female to improve the embryo recognition and prevent rejection. LIT can also down-regulate NK cell activation, improving the balance of TH-1 and TH-2 cells in the uterus. However, similar benefits can be achieved through IL therapy combined with corticosteroids. The use of LIT is prohibited in the United States.

Baby M's Story

My husband and I tried to grow our family for seven years, which included two years of IVF treatments. It has been nothing short of a tiresome and heartbreaking process (as it is for any family struggling with infertility).

After a few years without any success, we sought medical advice and began fertility treatment. I was placed on Clomid and, after three rounds, I suffered my first chemical pregnancy. We attended a local fertility clinic in 2017, where I was diagnosed with "unexplained infertility." We also became financially strained and were unable to continue with any fertility treatments. We were devastated and continued to try naturally without any success for the next three years.

In 2020, we were able to return to the local fertility clinic and underwent three rounds of IUI without any success. I decided I would give up because we could not afford the cost of IVF at any clinic in our area. I was at a loss and giving up hope.

One day, my friend introduced me to someone who had successfully completed an IVF cycle at a different clinic. She told me all about this clinic and sold me on scheduling a consultation. From the first consultation and every interaction thereafter, I was very pleased with the knowledge, kindness, and understanding nature of all of the medical staff. We were also able to afford the cost of IVF due to the affordability of ART treatments that this clinic graciously offers. We were so grateful.

We underwent retrieval and a fresh transfer, which unfortunately failed. Further testing via ReceptivaDx revealed that I had signs of endometriosis and a low AMH. I was treated for two months with Lupron Depot before my frozen embryo transfer. Unfortunately, this transfer also failed.

After two failed rounds of IVF, my husband and I fell on financial hardship yet again. I had a laparoscopy performed to determine if I had endometriosis, which resulted in the removal of endometriomas and one of my Fallopian tubes (which was blocked), and a diagnosis of stage 3 endometriosis. We went back to the clinic for a third round and spent the very last of our savings in hopes of bringing home our miracle. But, again, this cycle failed.

After this, the loved ones in our community, family, and Church raised funds to help us try again. We underwent another round of IVF and two more transfers, all of which failed and left us devastated.

We did not want to give up and were willing to fight through this to bring home our baby. We began to sell our possessions and home to afford further treatment, and then we went through another failed cycle of IVF.

Immunology testing took place next and we discovered that I had elevated NKC (Natural Killer Cells) and a possible APS (antiphospholipid syndrome) diagnosis. This means that my immune system was abnormally attacking proteins in my blood, which increased my risk of developing blood clots.

Eventually, it was recommended that my husband and I both transition to a carnivore (low inflammation) lifestyle and diet. I credit the transition as the "missing link" to receiving our little miracle. Additionally, I was placed on an immunologic protocol to suppress my immune system enough to accept a transferred embryo.

After just 74 days of following a strict carnivore lifestyle, I experienced the following results:

- My depression, painful periods, bloating, and cystic acne disappeared
- My hair grew back
- My psoriasis cleared up
- I felt stronger and able to lift heavier weights at the gym

My husband and I underwent another transfer of two day 5 embryos. We shared a prayer with the IVF clinic staff after the transfer was complete. For the first time through this entire process, I felt peace and confidence after the transfer because I knew we had done all we possibly could.

At the time of beta testing, I tested positive for a pregnancy! Our beautiful little girl was born on Easter Sunday 2023. I often find myself just sitting and staring at my baby in absolute awe of it all. God is Good.

I hope sharing my story helps others who are struggling to find answers feel that they are not alone. I also look forward to sharing my story with others in hopes of inspiring individuals and families on their fertility journeys to never give up on finding the right path that will bring home their little miracles.

Conclusions

The complex interaction between embryonic cells and the lining of the uterus plays a critical role in successful implantation. There are many causes of reproductive failure, including embryonic factors, uterine abnormalities, and immunologic implantation dysfunction. If you are experiencing reproductive failure, it is important to understand the causes and possible treatment options to improve your reproductive outcomes.

Chapter 10
Coping with Loss and Grief

The information in this chapter was contributed by Kendra A. Vargas, LCPC, PMH-C, owner/founder of Authentically You Psychotherapy.

Welcome to the chapter on loss and grief. This chapter may feel deeply personal and could evoke past and present emotions that remain difficult to process. Please read at a pace that feels right for you—this is emotionally weighted content, and it's okay to take breaks. My hope is that by the end of this chapter, you'll feel seen, supported, and validated. Grief is normal. It is real. And you are not alone.

Identifying grief can be challenging, especially when it's woven into the journey of trying to build a family. Many people struggle to comprehend the feelings they experience because grief is often complicated, confusing, and layered with mixed emotions that add further complexity. *Loss at any stage of a pregnancy can be absolutely devastating and the emotional impact is often underestimated.*

Grief is often overlooked, and many people do not realize that what they're experiencing is actually grief. After they begin the process of family planning and so many events unfold (e.g., miscarriage or failed transfer), they continue to push forward. This urgency, whether driven by a sense of mission or the ticking of a biological clock, can leave them with little time to pause and process their emotions. As a result, grief may go unacknowledged, even as it quietly shapes the emotional landscape of their journey.

We often associate grief with losing a loved one with whom you've shared memories and experiences. With the grief we are focusing on in this chapter, there typically aren't tangible memories and experiences, making it a unique and challenging emotional experience that is often misunderstood. This can make it harder to explain, harder to validate, and harder for others to understand.

This kind of grief is often invisible, especially to those who haven't experienced infertility or pregnancy loss. But that doesn't make it any less real. It deserves space, recognition, and care.

Recognizing Grief Associated with Pregnancy-Related Loss

As people grieve their pregnancy-related losses, they may experience a wide range of emotions, many of which may shift rapidly and feel overwhelming. If you are experiencing please consider reaching out to a support person or a licensed professional—you don't have to navigate this alone.

These emotions may arise individually or all at once, and they may ebb and flow over time. Grief is not linear—it's a deeply personal process that unfolds in its own rhythm. Common emotions that people experience as they grieve their pregnancy-related losses include:

- Sadness
- Self-blame ("Did I do something wrong?")
- Shock
- Denial
- Numbness
- Guilt (e.g., feeling guilt for not protecting the child)
- Inadequacy (doubt of their abilities, feeling flawed)
- Anger or resentment
- Isolation
- Emptiness
- Panic
- Jealousy
- Confusion

Causes of Grief and Loss in the Context of Family Planning

Grief and loss related to family planning can stem from one or more of the following experiences:

- Failing to conceive before receiving an infertility diagnosis (see Chapter 1)
- Receiving an infertility diagnosis (see Chapter 5)
- Experiencing a failed IUI or IVF cycle (see Chapter 9)
- Receiving a negative pregnancy test result
- Receiving a confirmed pregnancy loss (e.g., an ectopic pregnancy, miscarriage, missed miscarriage, or stillbirth)
- Terminating a pregnancy for medical reasons (TFMR)
- Inability to biologically create a child with your partner
- Disruptions in your family-building arrangements
- Choosing to end the family-planning process
- Experiencing the loss of the gestational carrier (surrogate) you were originally working with
- Beginning a pregnancy with twins and then experiencing a loss of one or both

While the type of loss that one experiences in these examples varies, grief is present in every single one of them. Let's take a closer look at some of the previously mentioned experiences and explore common emotions associated with them.

- **A failed IUI procedure.** IUI cycles are often performed month after month, so the time in between them is short. This leaves little time to process grief between attempts. Many people continue to push through failed cycles, which can be mentally draining. At the same time, their grief may be delayed or completely ignored.

    After multiple failed IUIs, transitioning to in vitro fertilization (IVF) can bring a mix of emotions. Some may feel mentally stronger from their previous experiences, while others may feel emotionally drained from the repeated grief they've already endured. Alternatively, they may be emotionally numb or have feelings of fear, excitement to try a new option, or nervousness.

- **A failed IVF cycle.** There are weeks (or even months) of exhaustive prep work (e.g., medication administration and monitoring) that must be completed leading up to an IVF cycle. So, waking up from the sedation after your egg retrieval and receiving the news that only a few or no eggs were retrieved can be devastating. Even those who go into an egg retrieval expecting poor results are often still hurt by this news.

  And, even if eggs are retrieved, there is no guarantee that they will fertilize and develop properly. In some situations, no embryos result from an IVF cycle, or no embryos are genetically normal and able to be transferred. There are various reasons why these events occur, but they can still cause a lot of confusion that usually sets in after the initial shock wears off.

  For those who experience one or more failed IVF cycles, questions may arise about the feasibility and worthiness of moving forward with another cycle. While there are many advancements in science and medicine that have made IVF more predictable, there are still many aspects of the process that are unknown, which can add additional stress and anxiety to the experience. Some unknowns surrounding a failed IVF cycle may include:

  - Your overall success rate
  - The number of cycles that it will take to get you to a point to move forward to a transfer
  - What emotions will show up throughout the process
  - Whether or not the side effects will be minimal or difficult to manage
  - How long the overall process will take

  When a cycle fails, those unknowns can amplify anxiety and self-blame. You might ask yourself questions like:

  - What's wrong with me?
  - Did I do something to cause this?
  - Is this the right treatment for me?

  There is loss here because you hoped for something that did not come to fruition, and it's necessary to grieve those unfulfilled expectations.

- **A negative pregnancy test.** Each cycle may carry anticipation, hope, and emotional buildup. A negative result is a loss—not just of a potential pregnancy, but of the joy, connection, and future you envisioned. For example, you might anticipate the joy you will feel when you see the positive pregnancy test or think about sharing the news with others.

Receiving a negative pregnancy result is a loss because *you grieve what you thought you might see:* a positive test and future that you might have been a step closer to. Whether you were the person planning to carry the pregnancy, a partner, or a surrogate, hearing that "it didn't work" can be gut-wrenching. This is grief.

- **A failed embryo transfer.** An embryo transfer often follows weeks of injections, monitoring, and emotional ups and downs. Additionally, the "two-week wait" following the transfer can be emotionally taxing, filled with hyper-awareness and cautious optimism.

    When a transfer fails, it's a loss—of time, energy, and emotional investment.

    Repeated failures can erode hope and increase feelings of helplessness. Even physical discomfort from injections adds to the emotional toll. Each failed transfer can feel like a setback, and when hope is reignited by new testing or procedures, another failure can reopen the wound.

    Transfers can fail for multiple reasons, and sometimes there are additional steps that can be taken, such as further testing or surgical procedures, that can potentially increase your chances of success (see Chapter 9). Completing these tests or procedures can re-instill a level of hope because the logical part of our brains sees that there's been a way to solve the problem and now feels new and fresh. People toggle between their emotional and logical brain compartments throughout this process, which can get exhausting over time. But when there's another failure after what was thought to be an identified reason, it can cause grief all over again.

- **Pregnancy loss.** *Loss at any stage of a pregnancy is real and matters deeply.*

  When you or the person carrying your baby sees a positive pregnancy test or ultrasound, it's common to form an instant connection with your baby because your future dreams start feeling closer to reality. This can happen even to those who are cautiously optimistic about their pregnancies. It's also very common to feel anxious when you see a positive pregnancy test or ultrasound because you have established a strong connection that you are very afraid to lose. This anxiety may arise if you or someone you know has experienced a miscarriage in the past. Regardless, a pregnancy loss is a traumatic experience because you are forced to break the connection that you have formed with your unborn baby and shift your plans and dreams for your future.

  Many people who have experienced pregnancy loss contemplate attempting another pregnancy. As much as they want to become pregnant again, they may fear facing another miscarriage or a failed attempt at pregnancy. This is especially true when there is no clear answer or explanation for a miscarriage, which makes trying again even more terrifying. Often, people try so hard to find answers that make them feel at ease about moving forward because it is difficult for them to cope with an explanation of "it just happened." Though 50–80 percent of people become pregnant following a miscarriage, there are higher rates of anxiety and depression that accompany pregnancies that follow a loss.

  Pregnancy loss can also shake your sense of identity. You may start asking yourself heavy questions, such as: "Who am I if I can't carry my baby?" or "Who am I if I can't become a parent?" Even though about 15–20 percent of pregnancies end in loss, the grief is personal and deeply felt. It's the loss of someone you imagined would be part of your life forever.

  Other complex emotions such as inadequacy, anger, sadness, guilt may also arise following a miscarriage.

> ### Sarah's Story
>
> *I went into my marriage knowing that I had PCOS, so we started trying to conceive right away knowing that it could take a little longer for us to get pregnant. After nine months of trying, we got our first positive pregnancy test, and it was the happiest day of our lives. We were so excited and immediately started planning what life would look like with a Spring baby.*
>
> *But, after a few weeks of joy, I noticed that I was bleeding after using the bathroom. I knew I had miscarried and I was instantly devastated. I grieved in a way that I didn't know I was capable of. I was full of so much sadness, anger, and confusion.*
>
> *If you would have told me at that point that the next few years would result in a successful pregnancy, two more pregnancy losses, and three years of trying for baby number two, I would have never believed you. I wouldn't have thought I could do it. But infertility has shown me the importance of taking care of and supporting myself and learning to navigate heavy emotions.*
>
> *I hope that my story can show someone who feels at their lowest of lows that we are all capable of navigating through this tough time. Even if it feels impossible, there is hope.*

Factors That Affect Grief Associated with Loss

As you can see, there are a variety of emotions that accompany grief and loss, and all of these emotions are valid. Grief comes in waves. It can hit you when you least expect it, its stages are sometimes chaotic and unpredictable, and it can often be isolating. Whatever you feel is a reflection of your experience, and it deserves space.

In addition to internal emotional responses, external factors can intensify grief and make it harder to process. Two of the most common are social factors and triggers.

- **Social factors**

    Social acceptance of pregnancy-related loss is often limited, especially when the loss occurs early or involves a failed treatment cycle. There's even less understanding when someone experiences loss through surrogacy, as the grief may be dismissed because they weren't physically carrying the child.

    The outside world often does not take into consideration all of the time and effort that went into getting to this point. People mean well and often struggle with what to say and how to show their support, but sometimes their words can be dismissive, hurtful, and invalidating. Have you heard any of these before?

    - "At least you can get pregnant!"
    - "Just try again!"
    - "Everything happens for a reason."
    - "Maybe it just wasn't meant to be."
    - "It will happen when the time is right."

    These statements, though often intended to comfort, can feel dismissive and isolating. They overlook the depth of your grief and the complexity of your journey. There's a hidden grief that many don't recognize or understand, and some may even impose timelines for when you should "move on" or "be over it."

- **Triggers**

    Triggers. Are. Everywhere. A trigger is anything that evokes a strong emotional response and brings you back to your loss. They can appear suddenly and without warning, reigniting grief and emotional pain. Common triggers include:

    - Pregnancy announcements
    - Birth of someone's baby
    - Commercials, tv shows, or movies
    - Seeing someone pregnant
    - Parks filled with children
    - Families at the beach
    - Holidays
    - Due dates or loss anniversaries
    - Seeing fertility medications or needles
    - Conversations about babies, pregnancies, or family
    - Questions about your journey
    - Menstruation
    - Social media posts of babies or children

Primary and Secondary Loss

When we talk about loss, we often focus on the primary loss—the event itself, such as a miscarriage, failed cycle, or the end of a family-building journey. But grief is rarely that simple. There are often secondary losses that accompany the primary one, and these can be just as impactful, even if they're harder to name or understand.

Secondary losses may include:

- Loss of faith or trust in your body, in medicine, or in the process
- Loss of income, especially if treatment costs or time off work are involved
- Loss of control over your timeline, your body, or your future
- Loss of dreams, hope, or the vision you had for your family
- Loss of identity, especially if parenthood was central to how you saw yourself
- Loss within relationships, including strain with friends, family, or romantic partners

These losses are layered, and they often interact with other life stressors like career demands, family conflict, or personal responsibilities. The emotional weight can feel overwhelming.

Hormonal changes after a miscarriage or the discontinuation of fertility medications can also significantly impact your mood and emotional regulation. If you live with a mental health condition, the emotional toll of loss may feel even heavier and more difficult to manage. These factors don't just add to grief—they can amplify it, making it harder to process and more isolating.

Grief is not just about what was lost. It's also about what was attached to that loss: your expectations, your identity, your relationships, and your future. Recognizing these secondary losses is a powerful step toward healing.

Coping with Grief and Loss in Family Planning

Grieving a pregnancy loss is a deeply personal experience. How someone copes depends on their unique circumstances, emotional history, and support system. There is no "right" way to grieve, but there are ways to support yourself through it.

- **Differentiate what is in your control versus what is out of your control.** Grief often brings a sense of helplessness. You may feel powerless over test results, treatment outcomes, or whether a pregnancy will occur. While many aspects of family planning are outside your control (e.g., the outcome of a test or cycle), identifying what is within your control can help reduce stress. You can control:
    - Your thoughts and feelings
    - Your behavior
    - What you choose to give energy to
    - How you speak to yourself
    - Your boundaries
    - Your choices
    - Your goals
    - Your decisions
    - How you choose to cope
- **Accept what has happened.** Acceptance doesn't mean approval. You can accept your reality while still feeling upset, disappointed, or angry.

    Many people resist acceptance, believing it means they're condoning what happened. But resisting reality often prolongs emotional suffering. So, let's talk about how to change that.

    In Dialectical Behavior Therapy (DBT), there's a skill called Radical Acceptance that can help reduce emotional suffering. Radically accepting what you've been through doesn't mean you like or agree with what happened. Instead, it's about acknowledging reality as it is and letting go of resistance so you can begin to heal.

    Change can also occur while working toward acceptance. For example, you can:
    - Radically accept your infertility diagnosis AND take steps to follow your fertility specialist's guidance.
    - Radically accept there's been an unexpected change in your family-building plan, AND explore your options and next steps.
    - Radically accept all emotions, even ones that feel complicated.

- **Grieve your loss(es).** Grief is unavoidable. Everyone grieves differently, and others may have opinions about how you "should" grieve. But your grief is yours. Allow yourself time, space, and grace.

  Understanding the five stages of grief (Kübler-Ross Model) can help normalize your experience. Keep in mind that these stages of grief are not linear, and some people may only experience some (or none) of the stages. Below are the five stages and how they may show up for you.
  - **Denial** serves to not overwhelm people with the intense emotions of a loss all at once. Denial and shock can help you to better pace your grief, which allows you to cope and survive through the grieving process. Examples of denial may include statements such as "My doctors are wrong" or "I'm fine" following a loss.
  - **Anger** is a necessary release when reality sets in. Keep in mind that you may project that anger onto others. Examples of anger may include statements such as "Why me?" and "This isn't fair."
  - **Bargaining** occurs when false hope comes into play and a person may be willing to do anything to get back to how they felt before their loss. Guilt and "what if" thinking often show up at this stage, and statements like "What if I ate healthier" or "What if I didn't take that long walk?" may surface. Individuals may also try to negotiate or make deals in their minds to reverse or alter the painful reality that they are facing.
  - **Depression**, which usually accompanies emptiness, isolation, loneliness, sadness, often presents at this stage. This is when reality has officially settled in and you realize that your experience is truly a loss.
  - **Acceptance** is the final stage of grief and occurs when you are learning how to move forward in your reality and live with your loss. This doesn't mean you'll never feel saddened by your loss. There will be moments of peace and sadness, but moving forward should hopefully feel less heavy.
- **Journaling.** Writing can be a powerful outlet for emotions you're not ready to share aloud. Journaling helps you process your thoughts, release tension, and track your healing journey.
- **Letter writing or a memorial service.** Some find comfort in writing a letter to the child they miscarried or to their future unborn child as a way to find a sense of closure. Writing can be very cathartic, so if you feel that is a way to release emotions or transition to your next phase of the process, this can be a very helpful tool.

Another way people seek solace or resolution in the face of their loss is by having a memorial service with their partner and/or loved ones. This service can be a powerful tool to utilize when going through the healing process. These services can offer closure, validation, and a sense of control in a time that feels chaotic.

- **Setting Boundaries**: Boundaries are the limits you put in place to protect your well-being and help you navigate the variety of emotions you may experience after your loss.

  They help you navigate conversations, social settings, and triggers after a loss.

Some examples of boundaries might include:

- Telling a friend or loved one limited information about the loss. You can tell them you are not ready to discuss the loss in detail, but that you want them to know about it and would like them to check in with you over the next week or so. If you are not comfortable answering questions, tell them to please not ask you specific questions right now, and let them know that you will share more information when you're ready. Consider your needs and limits when sharing your information, and be aware that sometimes people may not know how to support you. It may benefit you to say something like, "I would love for you to support me by _____."
- Limiting your social media exposure to avoid pregnancy announcements or family photos.
- Avoiding phone calls and instead communicating through texts or emails to control when and how you respond.
- Skipping events because you do not want to answer questions or talk to others as you grieve. This is especially true for triggering events such as baby showers.
- Setting physical boundaries around intimacy and physical contact as you recover.
- **Breathe**. These powerful tools can be practiced anytime to help reduce stress and bring you back to the present moment. Breathing regulates your nervous system and sends calming signals to your brain. Check in with yourself throughout the day and build in some breaks to focus on your breathing. Get into the habit of noticing your breath and what's happening within and around you. Here are a few breathing exercises that you can incorporate into your daily routine:

- Belly breathing: Sit or lie down in a comfortable position. Place one hand on your belly and the other on your chest. Next, slowly inhale deeply through your nose and feel your belly rise. Then, slowly exhale through your mouth and feel your belly fall. Repeat as needed, and tune into the sensations in your breath and body throughout the process.
- Box breathing: Inhale through your nose for a slow count of four (count in your mind), then hold your breath for a count of four. After that, exhale through your nose for a count of four, and finally hold your breath for a count of four before beginning again. Visualize tracing the sides of a box with each step—up, across, down, and back—creating a rhythm that calms and centers you.

- **Take a break.** Taking a break doesn't mean giving up—it means giving yourself space to breathe, reflect, and heal. Whether it's a pause from fertility treatments, decision-making, conversations, or social media, breaks can be restorative and clarifying. People often struggle with taking breaks because they want to continue moving forward and avoid "wasting any time." In some cases, the decision to take a break can actually increase stress and anxiety levels (which makes them ineffective), but breaks are rarely ever regretted and are often very beneficial.

    People take breaks for a variety of reasons, including:
    - You, your partner, or your surrogate have experienced a loss
    - You or anyone involved in the family-planning process is feeling drained and emotionally exhausted ("burnt out")
    - You are conflicted on what steps to take next in your journey.

    A break can help you process what you've been through, relieve pressure, and reconnect with your sense of self. It's important to discuss any treatment-related breaks with your doctor or therapist to ensure they align with your care plan.

- **Practice self-care.** Self-care is not just about spa days or vacations, it's about tending to your emotional, physical, and mental needs in everyday life. Everything discussed in this section—setting boundaries, breathing, taking breaks, grieving, asking for help—is a form of self-care.

    Other foundational self-care practices include:
    - Getting enough sleep
    - Moving your body in ways that feel good
    - Staying hydrated
    - Nourishing yourself with food
    - Creating space for joy, rest, and reflection

Self-care is not selfish, it's essential. Especially in the context of grief and family planning, it's a way to honor your experience and support your healing.

When to Seek Help

Anyone who has experienced loss related to family planning is likely to face emotional challenges throughout their journeys, including but not limited to:

- Depression
- Anxiety
- Post Traumatic Stress Disorder (PTSD)
- Stress (personal, relational, or marital)
- Grief
- Guilt and shame

If you have a mental health diagnosis and/or a family history of mental health conditions, you may be at a higher risk for developing a mental health condition following a loss. If you are not feeling like yourself or are experiencing any of the following for more than a few days, it may be time to talk to someone:

- A loss of interest in activities that you previously enjoyed
- Low, depressed mood (being in a funk you can't get out of)
- Intrusive thoughts about the loss
- Heightened stress, worry, or anxiety
- Sleep disturbances (too little or too much sleep)
- Flashbacks or nightmares about the loss
- Thoughts of suicide or death
- Appetite changes (not eating enough or eating too much)
- Difficulty concentrating or focusing
- Ongoing irritability
- Isolation
- Guilt and shame, especially self-blame for the loss

A licensed mental health professional can help you navigate these emotions. When searching for a therapist (e.g., counselor, psychologist, social worker), look for someone with experience in grief and loss, infertility, perinatal mental health, and trauma (if applicable to you).

Postpartum Support International is an international organization that supports individuals and families during pregnancy, loss, and postpartum challenges. It is also one of the few international certification programs for therapists to become certified in perinatal mental health through evidence-based training programs. Therapists with a PMH-C (Perinatal Mental Health Certification) have completed specialized training and ongoing education in the field of perinatal mental health. Therefore, working with someone with this certification is highly recommended.

There are various types of therapies available, including:

- **Individual therapy** is one-on-one therapy that provides you with a safe space to explore your emotions, process your loss, and develop coping strategies. You will feel heard, validated, and supported as you work through personal challenges and learn tools to manage your symptoms in your daily life. This is your space just for you.
- **Couples therapy** refers to therapy for you and your partner. Grief and loss as they relate to family planning can strain relationships. Couples therapy can help you and your partner learn how to support one another through this part of your journey. If you have been going through fertility treatments, or have had a loss or multiple losses, there are different emotions that arise for each of you individually that can sometimes be difficult to understand. Couples therapy helps partners:
    - Understand each other's boundaries and grieving styles
    - Improve communication
    - Hold space for one another
    - Rebuild an emotional connection
    - Navigate decisions together
- **Group therapy** involves attending group support sessions for pregnancy loss, fertility support, surrogacy loss or support, and more. These groups can help you to feel less isolated in your experience. There's something about being in a space with other people going through a similar experience as you that feels so validating. These can be safe spaces for you to heal, share your experiences, feel supported, learn from one another, and support others. Organizations like Postpartum Support International and RESOLVE offer free virtual and in-person groups, making this an accessible and impactful resource.

- **Medication management** refers to taking medications prescribed by your doctor to help manage depression, anxiety, or PTSD. Common options include antidepressants or anti-anxiety medications, many of which are safe for use during pregnancy and postpartum. Research shows that therapy combined with medication can be especially effective. If you're considering this option, speak with your healthcare provider to explore what's best for your needs.

Road to Rainbow

My husband and I were married in July 2016 and (naively) assumed that we would become pregnant right away. We got pregnant on our honeymoon and then had a miscarriage around six weeks. We were devastated, but also hopeful that we would become pregnant again quickly since the first pregnancy happened right away.

After a year of trying (with ovulation predictor kits, acupuncture, Chinese herbs, diets, etc.), we decided to go to a fertility clinic. I was diagnosed with diminished ovarian reserve (DOR) and instructed to begin an IVF cycle for fertility preservation (embryo banking).

I was crushed and felt like my womanhood had been given a death sentence.

We ended up with two genetically normal embryos after our first round, but they also found a mass on my ovary. I went to an oncologist, who suggested that I get the mass removed because it could be (or become) cancerous. Though the mass was fortunately benign, they had to remove my ovary and Fallopian tube during the procedure.

After we completed two more rounds of IVF, we ended up with a grand total of six normal embryos in storage. When the time came to transfer them, we were so hopeful and optimistic, thinking that the worst was behind us. Well, it wasn't.

After three failed transfers, the doctor said that we "just had bad luck." I completed a recurrent pregnancy loss panel, sonohysterogram, hysteroscopy, and uterine biopsy, but everything came back as normal. There was no explanation as to why three perfect embryos were not implanting into a perfect uterus.

I tried a different protocol for our fourth transfer, which resulted in a positive pregnancy. But we quickly found ourselves in "beta Hell" and learned that we were having a missed miscarriage. I underwent a Manual Vacuum Aspiration (MVA), and then we sought a new clinic.

The new clinic suggested we do another hysteroscopy to make sure that my uterine lining was clear after my MVA procedure. They discovered scar tissue on my uterus, which needed to be cleared up before we could do another transfer.

I know that scar tissue alone can cause infertility, so I was not optimistic about our chances. While waiting for the scar tissue to resolve, we did another egg retrieval and ended up with four normal embryos. We also applied to a surrogacy agency for a gestational carrier (GC). However, there was an eight to ten month wait for a GC, and I was starting to feel like I could not take another loss in my own body. So, we waited.

Another hysteroscopy was performed five months later, which revealed that the scar tissue was still in my uterus. At this point, we were only three months away from being matched with a GC. I finally came to terms with the fact that I was not going to be able to carry or breastfeed my baby, but I was okay with that if it meant that I could be a mom.

My uterus cleared up when we were two weeks away from being matched with a GC. Our doctor suggested that we try one more transfer, and I agreed, thinking that we could at least say we tried everything one last time before moving on to a GC.

That "one last time" led to our sweet rainbow baby, Makena.

After Makena was born, I decided to write her a book titled Road to Rainbow, which described our journey and how hard we fought to get to her. While reading the book, I realized that the roadblocks on the way to the rainbow could represent other obstacles that people must overcome to get to their rainbow babies and I knew that others could relate to the story.

We want to share our joy, be honest about our struggles, and give hope to the one in six couples that are walking their own "road to rainbow."

Conclusions

Grief and loss, especially in the context of family building, bring forth complex, multilayered emotions that may be difficult to understand, both for yourself and for those around you. These emotions are valid, even when they feel messy or contradictory.

Healing begins with the courage to acknowledge, accept, and honor your experience. There is no single path through grief, and no timeline that must be followed. With time, care, and support, you can learn how to move forward. But remember: grief is not linear. It may ebb and flow, rise unexpectedly, or feel quiet for long stretches. That's okay.

Be patient with yourself. Healing is not a destination—it's a journey. And you are not alone.

"What we once enjoyed and deeply loved we can never lose, for all that we love deeply becomes part of us." —Helen Keller

Chapter 11
Optimizing Reproductive Health

The information in this chapter was contributed by Jennifer McLeland, MD, MBA, a board-certified OB/GYN.

Introduction

Your reproductive health is shaped by a complex interplay of hormones, immune function, genetics, lifestyle choices, and environmental exposures. A problem in one area can affect others, impacting your ability to conceive or maintain a healthy pregnancy. Therefore, it's important to understand all of the factors that can influence your reproductive health so you can create a proactive and holistic strategy to optimize your fertility outcomes. Research suggests that it may take approximately 90 days to begin seeing measurable changes in both male and female fertility after implementing lifestyle and medical interventions. Here are some examples of factors that can influence your reproductive health:

- **Hormonal balance**: Healthy levels of estrogen, progesterone, testosterone, luteinizing hormone (LH), and follicle-stimulating hormone (FSH) are crucial for a normal for regular menstrual cycles and ovulation in females, and healthy sperm production and sexual function in males.
- **Fallopian tube health**: The fallopian tubes act as pathways for the egg, sperm, and embryo. Thus, they must remain open and functional. Blockages or damage from previous infections or surgery can impair these processes.

- **Uterine health**: A healthy uterus supports embryo implantation and pregnancy. Conditions like endometrial polyps, fibroids, scar tissue, and endometriosis can affect fertility.

- **Egg quantity and quality**: Recall from Chapter 3 that women are born with all the eggs that they will ever have, and egg number and quality decline over time. Eggs are affected by exposure to environmental toxins, diet, and stress. Other factors, such as genetics, can also impact egg quantity and quality.

- **Sperm production**: Males need a sufficient number of motile, normal-looking sperm for ideal fertility. Many factors, such as lifestyle choices, environmental exposures, medical conditions, and medications, can influence sperm production.

- **Sexually transmitted infections (STIs)**: Some STIs like gonorrhea and chlamydia can cause scarring and damage to the reproductive organs of both males and females that can lead to difficulties with fertility.

- **Lifestyle choices**: This is one of the most crucial (and most modifiable) aspects of reproductive health. Key habits such as maintaining a healthy weight, eating a balanced diet, engaging in regular physical activity, avoiding smoking and excessive alcohol intake, and managing stress all contribute to better overall reproductive health.

- **Oxidative stress**: This occurs when there's an imbalance between the production of harmful molecules called reactive oxygen species (ROS) and the body's ability to neutralize them with antioxidants. Excessive ROS can damage cellular components like DNA and proteins, and high levels can cause infertility.

Optimizing Female Fertility

Female fertility depends on a delicate interplay between hormonal balance, egg health, and overall well-being. While the cause of infertility remains unknown for some, many individuals can find improvements through dietary and lifestyle changes. Not every factor is within your control, but focusing on what is can make a meaningful difference. However, you should always consult with a healthcare professional before making any decisions about your health.

- **Maintain a healthy diet**: The food choices we make can significantly impact our fertility. Specific nutrients and dietary patterns can help balance hormone levels, reduce oxidative stress, and prevent inflammation. A female fertility approach often emphasizes a diet rich in antioxidants, similar to the popular Mediterranean diet. If you're unsure about making dietary changes for fertility, consulting a registered dietitian or fertility specialist can be helpful for personalized guidance.

- Things to avoid:
  - Focus on limiting simple processed carbohydrates, such as white sugar and high-fructose corn syrup, as studies suggest they may be linked to fertility issues. Simple carbohydrates, like those found in white bread, sugary drinks and snacks, and pasta, can cause rapid spikes in blood sugar and insulin levels, which can lead to insulin resistance, disrupt hormonal balance, impair ovulation, and potentially harm egg quality.
  - Low-fat dairy products *may* not be ideal for female fertility. Low-fat dairy products are often more processed to maintain their consistency once the fat is removed, and they have a different hormonal content than their full-fat counterparts. Some studies have found that the consumption of low-fat dairy has been shown to disrupt ovulation.[1] If dairy products are an integral part of your diet, moderate consumption of full-fat dairy products (e.g., whole milk, Greek yogurt, cheese) might be recommended.
  - Ultra-processed trans-fats are pro-inflammatory and can cause hormonal imbalances, insulin resistance, and cellular inflammation that can damage egg quality. Limiting or avoiding processed foods that contain trans-fats such as baked goods (cookies, cakes), margarine, nondairy coffee creamers, processed meats (hot dogs, deli meats), and fried foods (french fries, fried chicken) may improve your reproductive health. You can also supplement naturally occurring, unhydrogenated vegetable oils (canola, safflower, sunflower, olive oil) for cooking and baking.
  - Pesticides and Bisphenol A (BPA) contaminate food indirectly. Pesticides infiltrate fruits, vegetables, meat, and fish through water sources, while BPA leaches from food packaging like cans. Both act as xenoestrogens, mimicking estrogen in the body. Exposure can lead to hormonal imbalances, irregular periods or anovulation, reduced egg quality, and increased risk of miscarriage or pregnancy complications. While complete avoidance is impossible, strategies to reduce exposure include choosing organic foods to minimize pesticide residues (Check out the EWG's Dirty Dozen[2] and Clean Fifteen[3]), avoiding plastics (especially those with BPA), opting for glass or stainless steel, and filtering drinking water.

- Things to incorporate
    - Healthy fats, including omega-3 fatty acids (such as those found in wild-caught fish like salmon), certain oils (extra virgin olive oil), nuts (walnuts), avocados, and seeds (flaxseeds, chia seeds) can reduce oxidative stress, enhance egg quality, help regulate hormones necessary for ovulation, and improve blood flow to the uterus. Omega-3 fatty acids are particularly renowned for their anti-inflammatory properties, helping to create a healthier environment in the body and reproductive system.
    - Complex carbohydrates, such as whole grains (brown rice, quinoa, whole wheat bread and pasta, and oats), legumes, and vegetables, are digested slower and cause a gradual rise in blood sugar levels (thus, not causing spikes in insulin levels) compared to simple carbohydrates. They are good for your diet in moderation and should not be eliminated from your diet, unless under the direction of your doctor, when pursuing fertility. They are typically nutrient dense and have antioxidant and anti-inflammatory properties.
    - Plant-based protein sources, such as quinoa and lentils, have been linked to improved ovulation rates over animal-based protein sources. These foods are rich in fiber, antioxidants, and other nutrients such as folate, iron (lentils), and zinc (quinoa), which are important for fertility and future pregnancy.
    - Packed with antioxidants, fruits and vegetables are crucial for a balanced fertility diet. Leafy greens like spinach (spinach, kale, broccoli) and citrus fruits (oranges, lemons, grapefruits) are rich in folate, which is crucial for both fertility and early pregnancy development. They also provide potassium and calcium. Berries (blueberries, raspberries, strawberries), full of antioxidants and anti-inflammatory nutrients, support your ovaries. While they contain simple carbohydrates, the accompanying fiber helps regulate blood sugar and insulin levels.
- **Limit alcohol consumption**: Excessive alcohol can disrupt hormone balance, affect menstrual cycles, and impair fertility. Alcohol intake should be limited to one to two drinks per week. It is important to note that no safe amount of alcohol for pregnancy has been established, so it should be avoided entirely if pregnancy is possible.
- **Drink plenty of water**: Adequate water intake helps regulate reproductive hormones, promotes blood flow to the ovaries and uterus, assists with the removal of toxins and waste within the body, and promotes healthy cervical mucus production. In general, it's

recommended that women consume at least eight to ten cups of water daily, adjusting based on individual needs and circumstances. Pale yellow urine is a good indicator of adequate hydration.

- **Quit smoking**: Smoking accelerates egg loss, increases the risk of early menopause, and impairs the uterus's ability to support implantation. It also raises the risk of low birth weight and other complications. Quitting is one of the most impactful steps you can take for your reproductive and overall health.

- **Moderate caffeine intake**: High caffeine intake has been associated with delayed conception in some studies. A moderate amount (such as one cup of coffee or tea per day) is generally considered safe, but always follow your healthcare provider's guidance.

- **Reduce stress**: Chronic stress can interfere with ovulation and hormonal balance. Practices like meditation, journaling, deep breathing, or simply carving out quiet time can help decrease stress.

- **Get enough sleep**: Sleep is essential for hormone production and ovulatory health. Strive for 7–8 hours of restful sleep each night. Irregular sleep patterns may also disrupt reproductive rhythms.

- **Exercise**: Physical activity can improve fertility and pregnancy outcomes. However, extremes—either too much or too little—can be counterproductive. Choose movement that feels sustainable and nourishing, and consult your doctor if you're unsure what's best for your body.

- **Maintain a healthy weight**: Body mass index (BMI) influences egg quality, uterine lining health, and treatment outcomes. The most pronounced effects are typically at the extremes of the BMI spectrum. Obesity can lead to anovulation and reduced conception rates, while being underweight may cause hormonal disruptions that can affect ovulation.[4,5] The takeaway? Aim for a normal weight, if possible. Even modest weight changes can improve your fertility. Talk with your provider about safe strategies tailored to your individual needs.

- **Consider supplements** (but talk with your healthcare provider first!): While supplements can play a supportive role in your fertility, a balanced diet is the foundation. Our bodies are better at absorbing nutrients from whole foods. The one exception is folate, where supplementation (of folic acid) is often recommended to ensure adequate intake.

- Folate (folic acid) is crucial for cell division and neural tube development. Since neural tube formation begins early, folic acid is recommended *before* conception. Aim for a daily supplement containing 800 mcg, which is often included in prenatal vitamins (but always check the label).
- Choline support early neural development. Consider including a supplement containing at least 450 mg of choline daily when trying to conceive.
- Vitamin D helps reduce inflammation and supports reproductive health. Consider getting your vitamin D levels checked by a doctor to determine how much you should take. If testing is not readily available, a suggested starting point of 2,000 IU per day can be discussed with your healthcare provider.
- Coenzyme Q10 (CoQ10) is a nutrient found in nearly every cell in the body, including within the eggs. It acts as an antioxidant and reduces oxidative stress. It also supports mitochondrial (energy) function (and eggs have a lot of mitochondria!). A supplement containing 200 mg of ubiquinol can be added to your routine.

- **Take a prenatal vitamin**: Many prenatal vitamins already include essential antioxidants like vitamins E and C, which are also recommended in your diet. When considering additional supplements, be cautious as they aren't regulated by the FDA and may contain undeclared ingredients. Look for options with third-party testing and transparent labeling, avoiding those with vague "other ingredients".

Optimizing Male Fertility

Male fertility is often underrepresented in reproductive health conversations. However, according to the National Institute of Child Health and Human Development, male factors contribute to at least one-third of all infertility cases. Semen quality—particularly sperm count, motility, and morphology—is the primary predictor of male fertility, and research shows it has been declining globally.[6] There are many possible reasons for this decline, such as a change in lifestyle habits, smoking, alcohol intake, weight, physical activity, and diet.

The good news is that lifestyle changes can significantly improve semen quality, impacting your chances of conceiving. Here are some ways to optimize male fertility (after consulting with a healthcare provider!):

- **Maintain a healthy diet**:[7] A nutrient-dense diet supports hormonal health and protects sperm from oxidative stress. Consider consulting a fertility specialist or registered dietitian for personalized guidance.
  - Things to avoid:
    - Processed meats (bacon, sausage, ham, jerky, hot dogs, deli meats) may negatively impact sperm morphology,[8] but red meat or overall meat intake do not seem to have the same impact. However, this doesn't justify a "meat-only" diet. Maintain healthy portions and choose high-quality meats whenever possible.
    - Trans fats (found in fried foods and processed snacks) can lower testosterone, reduce sperm count and motility, and impair morphology.[9] See the section above for a list of common foods that contain trans-fats.
    - Xenoestrogens from pesticides or BPA that leach into food can disrupt testosterone production and impair sperm quality (count, motility, morphology). Studies have linked higher pesticide residue intake in foods to lower sperm counts and fewer normal sperm, and BPA has been associated with increased levels of sperm DNA damage.[10]
    - Full-fat dairy products (whole milk, cream, and high-fat cheeses) have been linked to reduced sperm motility and abnormal morphology. Opting for lower-fat alternatives is recommended.[11]
    - Mercury can damage sperm DNA. When possible, limit or avoid high-mercury fish (shark, swordfish, king mackerel) and opt for low-mercury options (salmon, sardines, shrimp, and light canned tuna).
  - Things to incorporate:
    - Healthy fats (see list above) may support hormone production, reduce inflammation, and improve sperm health. Studies suggest that eating fish rich in omega-3 fatty acids may reduce oxidative stress and improve sperm quality, possibly due to their anti-inflammatory properties. However, omega-3 supplements, even those derived from fish, haven't shown the same benefit. Interestingly, men who consume more fish tend to have higher sperm counts and normal sperm morphology. When choosing fish, it's important to select varieties with lower mercury levels like salmon.
    - Fruits and vegetables, especially those rich in color, are packed with nutrients and antioxidants (like vitamins B, C, and E) that support sperm health. Some standouts include:

- Dark leafy greens like spinach and kale are rich in folate (vitamin B9), an important antioxidant that can protect sperm from damage.
- Berries are rich in vitamin C and antioxidants that can protect sperm from oxidative stress and DNA damage.
- Tomatoes are a source of lycopene, folate, and vitamin C, all of which support sperm health.
- Tree nuts, especially walnuts and Brazil nuts, have been shown to improve sperm motility. Walnuts are rich in omega-3 fatty acids, which have anti-inflammatory properties, and in a small study showed that consumption may improve motility and morphology.[12] There are not a lot of studies that talk about Brazil nuts, but they are known to be rich in selenium, an antioxidant that can be very beneficial to sperm cell production.
- Lean proteins (salmon, tuna, oysters, poultry, eggs) provide essential amino acids, the building blocks for sperm cells, and other vital nutrients like zinc, selenium, and vitamin B12.
- Complex carbohydrates (see list above) provide sustained energy, help regulate blood sugar, and are a good source of vital minerals (zinc, selenium, magnesium) that support sperm production and health.

- **Limit alcohol consumption**: Heavy drinking can disrupt hormonal balance, impacting testosterone and estrogen levels. This imbalance may lead to reduced semen volume, lower sperm count, poor motility, and abnormal morphology.[13] Alcohol can also increase oxidative stress, which can damage sperm cells. For optimal fertility, limit alcohol to occasional drinks or avoid it altogether when trying to conceive.

- **Stay hydrated**: Adequate water intake can help improve semen volume and sperm quality, regulate hormone levels, reduce oxidative stress, and remove toxins and waste from the body. Aim for 8–10 cups of water daily unless otherwise advised by your healthcare provider.

- **Quit smoking**: Smoking's negative effects on health are widely understood, and that includes its impact on fertility. Studies show smoking (tobacco, marijuana, vaping) reduces sperm quality, impacting concentration, motility, and morphology. It can also disrupt male hormone levels and may impair sperm production. Quitting smoking may be one of the most impactful decisions for improving male fertility.[14]

- **Moderate caffeine consumption**: High caffeine intake may alter hormone levels and impact sperm quality, possibly through DNA damage[15]. Moderate consumption (such as one cup of coffee or tea per day) is generally considered safe.
- **Manage stress**: Chronic stress can disrupt testosterone production, reduce sperm quality, increase oxidative stress, and contribute to sexual dysfunction. Mindfulness, therapy, journaling, and regular relaxation can help restore hormonal balance and reduce stress.
- **Prioritize sleep**: Regular sleep and a healthy circadian rhythm are essential for cellular repair, hormonal regulation, and overall health. Disrupted sleep can increase oxidative stress, which can negatively impact sperm quality. Aim for 7–8 hours of sleep nightly and get sunlight exposure during the day to support your circadian rhythm.
- **Exercise**: Moderate exercise is crucial for overall health, including your heart, mood, and fertility. While moderate exercise can improve sperm quality (both count and motility), avoid excessive workouts, hot environments that raise your body temperature excessively (like hot yoga), and activities that apply pressure to the testicles (e.g., prolonged cycling). Importantly, using anabolic steroids or testosterone supplements can significantly and sometimes permanently harm sperm production.
- **Maintain a healthy weight**: Obesity is associated with reduced sperm quality (including increased DNA fragmentation), hormonal imbalances, oxidative stress, and chronic inflammation. Even modest weight loss can improve fertility outcomes.
- **Limit heat exposure to the testicles**: Sperm production requires a cooler environment in the testicles, so prolonged heat near the testicles can increase oxidative stress and impair sperm production and quality. Common heat sources include hot tubs, saunas, tight-fitting clothing and underwear, and laptops.
- **Consider a CoQ10 supplement** (after talking with a healthcare provider!): Coenzyme Q10 (CoQ10), a vitamin-like substance and powerful antioxidant, plays a vital role in cellular energy production, especially in sperm cells. Research suggests CoQ10 supplementation can benefit male fertility by improving sperm quality and reducing oxidative stress.

Toxic Environmental Exposures and Fertility

Environmental toxins pose a significant, and often invisible, threat to both male and female fertility. While complete avoidance is impossible, you can take steps to limit your exposure and improve your fertility and overall health. Common environmental toxins include endocrine-disrupting chemicals (EDCs), heavy metals, air pollution, and radiation.

Endocrine Disrupting Chemicals

- Endocrine-disrupting chemicals (EDCs) are substances that can mimic natural hormones like estrogen and testosterone, block their production, or alter how the body uses them. This can disrupt the delicate hormonal balance required for normal reproductive function.

  These chemicals are widely found in everyday items like food containers, some cosmetics, cleaning products, pesticides, and plastics. Reducing contact with EDCs can have a positive impact on your reproductive health.

  In men, EDCs may lower sperm count, reduce motility, and cause abnormal morphology, leading to decreased fertility. In women, EDCs can:

  - reduce ovarian reserve (the number of eggs in the ovaries), follicle development, and egg quality.
  - disrupt ovulation and menstrual cycles, potentially causing anovulation and irregular menstrual cycles.
  - Impair endometrial receptivity (how receptive the uterine lining is to an embryo), increasing the risk of implantation failure and miscarriage.

Common examples of EDCs include:
- **Bisphenol-A (BPA)**: Found in some plastics and food packaging, BPA may disrupt estrogen, testosterone, and thyroid hormones. Studies have linked BPA exposure to lower sperm and egg quality, reduced embryo development in IVF, and lower pregnancy rates. To minimize exposure, consider avoiding plastics, especially when heating food. Opt for glass or stainless steel containers when possible.
- **Per- and polyfluoroalkyl substances (PFAS)**: These "forever chemicals" are found in everyday items like food wrappers, non-stick

cookware, and some cosmetics and clothing. They may reduce sperm quality, disrupt ovarian reserve, and affect hormone production.

Here are some simple steps you can take to avoid PFAS:

- Choose stainless steel or cast iron cookware over non-stick versions.
- Avoid handling receipts and opt for digital options whenever possible.
- Wash all fruits and vegetables thoroughly before consumption.
- Filter your drinking water if it's contaminated.
- Opt for "PFAS-free" or "PFOA-free" and "PFOS-free" products in cosmetics, personal care items, and clothing.
- Avoid stain-resistant carpets and furniture, and vacuum regularly to minimize dust containing PFAS particles.

- **Phthalates**: Found in plastics, vinyl, cleaning products, and personal care items, phthalates are linked to cell damage, lower egg and sperm quality, and reduced testosterone levels. You can minimize exposure by choosing fragrance-free cleaning products, detergents, soaps, and hygiene products.

- **Pesticides** come from agriculture (herbicides like atrazine, insecticides like DDT), contaminated food, water, and soil. They can disrupt the endocrine system, impacting ovarian function and sperm quality. They can also increase the risk of implantation failure and miscarriage. Exposure can be minimized by choosing organic fruits and vegetables, washing and peeling produce, and filtering your drinking water.

Heavy Metals[16]

While heavy metals are found naturally in our environment, our exposure risk increases through certain workplace exposures and our food and water systems. Heavy metals can build up in our organs and tissues (including the ovaries[17] and testes) and induce oxidative stress. Toxic heavy metals, such as arsenic, lead, mercury, and cadmium, have been linked to decreased IVF success rates[18] and impaired sperm and egg quality.[19] In addition, these heavy metals have been shown to disrupt the endocrine system, which can impact the menstrual cycle and fertility. Lead and other heavy metals have also been associated with increased risks of miscarriage, stillbirth, and birth defects.

- **Lead** has fallen out of routine use in the United States since the 1970s. However, it still lingers in older homes (paint, pipes) and imported cosmetics.

Lead can affect male fertility by impacting sperm viability, motility, morphology, and DNA integrity. In women, lead can disrupt menstrual cycles, delay conception, alter hormone levels, and increase the risk of gestational hypertension, preterm birth, low birth weight, and miscarriage.[20]

You can decrease your exposure by taking proper safety precautions when remodeling homes built prior to 1978, avoiding drinking water from outdated plumbing, checking labels on imported cosmetics[21] (especially certain types of eyeliners), and ensuring that all precautions are in place if you have a high risk of exposure at your job.

- **Mercury** is a toxic heavy metal and neurotoxin that can be found in agricultural and manufacturing waste (mines and incineration plants), thermometers, batteries, pesticides, and dental products.[22]

  One form of mercury, methylmercury, can freely cross the placenta and increase the risk of cerebral palsy, mental retardation, and other neurological conditions in the developing fetus. It is important to remember that mercury accumulates in your tissues long before you become pregnant. In males, mercury can damage sperm DNA, reduce motility, and cause abnormal sperm morphology.[23]

  In regards to female fertility, mercury is thought to cause menstrual and hormonal disruption and can lead to poor reproductive outcomes.

  If you have the potential for workplace exposure to mercury, always wear proper protective gear. Also, avoid high-mercury fish and products.

- **Cadmium** can be found in rechargeable batteries, some fertilizers, paint, plastics, cigarette smoke (including e-cigarettes), and many foods grown in contaminated soil. In addition, occupational exposure can be significant for those involved in the making of cadmium products, welders, miners, smelters, and battery manufacturers.

  Cadmium affects male fertility by decreasing semen quality (especially motility), impairing sperm production, and disrupting hormone balance.[24]

  Cadmium affects female fertility by disrupting ovulation and implantation. It can also increase the risk of miscarriage and pregnancy complications like preterm birth.[25]

  Decrease your exposure by avoiding smoking and secondhand smoke, eating a healthy balanced diet, and using appropriate protective equipment if your occupation increases your exposure risk.

Air Pollution

Air pollution is an ongoing health concern for most of the world. Studies have shown that individuals living in areas with slightly higher levels of small particle pollution had their risk of fertility issues increased by as much as 20 percent. Air pollution can trigger oxidative stress and inflammation, reduce egg quality and ovarian reserve,[26] disrupt hormone balances, interfere with ovulation, and reduce sperm count and quality. It has been difficult to pinpoint the exact pollutant(s) causing these problems, though.

Here are some ways to avoid major sources of outdoor air pollution:

- Limit time outdoors, especially strenuous activity, on poor air quality days
- Reduce time on heavily trafficked roads
- Avoid rush hour if you commute
- Keep windows closed near busy roads[27]

Here are some ways to avoid major sources of indoor air pollution:

- Avoid exposure to tobacco smoke
- Limit use of indoor fireplaces
- Use an exhaust fan when cooking
- Consider purchasing a HEPA air filter for your home
- Maintain a diet rich in Omega-3 fatty acids and other antioxidants, as they may counteract some of the harmful effects of air pollution

Radiation

Radiation exposure can harm reproductive tissues and cells. Non-ionizing radiation is low-energy electromagnetic radiation that is found in many everyday devices (e.g., cell phones, Wi-Fi, laptops, microwaves) and natural resources. It has enough energy to make atoms and molecules vibrate or move, but not enough to strip electrons from them. Several studies have shown that non-iodizing radiation can harm ovarian and endometrial tissue in females,[28] as well as sperm health (motility, morphology, and count) in males[29]. Prolonged exposure, especially near the reproductive organs, should be limited if possible.

Ionizing radiation includes X-rays and radioactive particles used in medicine, manufacturing, and electric power production. This type of radiation is known to cause reproductive issues and can even cause birth defects.

High-risk occupations include flight attendants and airline workers such as pilots, healthcare and veterinary workers (especially those exposed to radioactive chemicals, fluoroscopy procedures, and X-ray machines), certain industrial workers, and certain laboratory technicians. Exposure to this type of radiation should be regulated in the workplace, and policies should be in place for workers that are pregnant. If you are pregnant or trying to conceive, consider speaking with your supervisor or radiation safety officer to ensure proper protections are in place.

Conclusions

There are many lifestyle factors that can influence your fertility, and making even minor changes can have lasting impacts on your fertility outcomes. Remember: Small changes add up! Try not to stress about the things you cannot change and not be overwhelmed by the harmful things in our environment. Start by making a few small, manageable and gradually incorporate more into your routine. And it's okay that you can't do everything all at once! Awareness is the first step toward protecting your fertility and overall health.

Chapter 12
Third-Party Reproduction

This chapter contains contributions from various professionals.

Introduction to Third-Party Reproduction

The information in this section was contributed by Cynthia Lim, director of marketing at Donor Concierge.

Third-party (donor-assisted) reproduction involves a person or couple (the intended parent(s)) receiving help from another individual (the third party) to achieve a healthy pregnancy. There are four main types of third-party reproduction:

- Sperm donors (known or non-identified)
- Egg donors (known or non-identified)
- Embryo donors (known or non-identified)
- Gestational carriers (surrogates who carry a pregnancy but are not genetically related to the fetus)

Third-party reproduction is most commonly pursued when one or either parent cannot conceive or carry a pregnancy using their own eggs, sperm, or uterus. However, there are many reasons why one might consider the use of third-party reproduction, including:

- Same-sex male couples or single male parents require donor eggs and a gestational carrier.
- Lesbian couples or single female parents require donor sperm.

- Males with absent or abnormal sperm production or other reproductive conditions may require donor sperm.
- Females with egg quality concerns, low ovarian reserve, or other reproductive conditions may require donor eggs.
- Couples who have failed to create viable embryos using their own gametes (eggs or sperm) may require donor gametes or embryos.
- Females who have had multiple failed transfers of good-quality embryos may require a gestational carrier.
- One or both parents may have a genetic condition that could cause harm to their offspring. In these cases, donor eggs, sperm, or embryos may be required.
- Lesbian couples may elect to undergo reciprocal IVF, in which one partner carries the pregnancy of a baby created with the other partner's egg, and vice versa.
- Other personal or medical reasons, including age-related fertility decline, cancer treatment history, or personal choice.

When to Consider Third-Party Reproduction

There is no universal timeline for when someone should consider third-party reproduction. This is a deeply personal decision that requires time and thought.

For some, the need is clear before fertility treatment begins. For example, same-sex couples or single parents know that they will require third-party reproduction (donor eggs and/or sperm) for fertilization to occur. Same-sex male couples know they will require a gestational carrier since neither partner has a uterus. And certain medical conditions may also warrant a need for third-party reproduction.

For others, the decision to use third-party reproduction is not based on anatomical factors and is usually not considered or recommended until after multiple failed attempts to conceive or carry a pregnancy.

Coping with Third-Party Reproduction

For some individuals and couples, the decision to pursue third-party reproduction is straightforward—often driven by anatomical or medical necessity. In these cases, the emotional impact may be minimal.

For others, the decision to use of third-party reproduction can trigger many emotions. Common emotional responses include:

- **Grief**. One or both parents may mourn the loss of a genetic connection to their child.
- **Blame**. It's common to internalize feelings of failure or guilt when fertility treatments are unsuccessful.
- **Relief**. After repeated setbacks, third-party reproduction may offer renewed hope and a sense of possibility.
- **Fear and anxiety**. The process can feel overwhelming, especially when navigating unfamiliar territory or facing societal stigma.
- **Indifference**. Not everyone experiences intense emotions—and that's okay too. Emotional responses vary widely.

Because this journey can be emotionally layered, speaking with a mental health professional (especially one familiar with fertility and family-building) can offer you a safe space to process your grief and emotions.

Other Considerations

Third-party reproduction opens doors to parenthood for many who cannot conceive through traditional means. It's a deeply personal journey, and there's no "right" way to approach it. Here are some ways to support yourself along the way:

- **Take it one step at a time.** Looking only at the entire process can be overwhelming, so try to break it down into manageable steps. It's important that you feel confident in your decisions every step of the way, so give yourself permission to pause and reflect as needed.
- **Do your research.** There is a lot of information available regarding third-party reproduction. Take some time to learn the terminology, understand your options, and explore the legal, ethical, and emotional dimensions of third-party reproduction so you can make informed decisions regarding your care.
- **Consult multiple clinics.** Each clinic may have different protocols, donor programs, and support services. Exploring your options helps you find the best fit for your needs.

- **Advocate for yourself.** As an intended parent, your voice matters. Ask questions, seek second opinions, and use available resources to make informed decisions.

> ### Emma's Story
>
> *Growing up, I always knew that I was donor conceived, and it was something that my family talked about openly. My parents struggled with infertility for six years and had almost given up hope of having children when they decided to try using a donor.*
>
> *After many attempts and a lot of money, I was finally born, and my parents went on to have ICSI twins two years later. Being a donor child has never been a negative experience for me. I have always felt like a full and equal member of my family, and my donor conception has never been a source of conflict or tension. In fact, my parents' openness and honesty about my conception has helped me feel comfortable and secure in my identity.*
>
> *As I got older, I started to share my story more widely, and I realized that there was a real need for positive donor-conceived narratives. Many of the stories I found online were negative and heartbreaking, and I wanted to share a different perspective. That's why I started my blog and wrote a book about our family's story. For me, anonymity has never been an issue, and I have never felt a need to connect with my donor or half-siblings. However, I recognize that everyone's experience is different, and some people may feel differently. That's why it's important to share our stories and perspectives without judgment.*
>
> *Overall, I believe that donor conception is an important option for anyone who may be struggling with infertility. It has allowed countless families to have children and build the families they have always dreamed of. My advice to parents of donor-conceived children is to be open and honest about their child's conception from an early age. By doing so, you can help your child feel secure and loved and avoid any unnecessary confusion or conflict later on.*

Donor Sperm Information

The following information was provided by Alyse Mencias, MS, former Clinic Relations Manager at Seattle Sperm Bank.

Sperm donation is a process in which a male provides sperm to help individuals or couples conceive through fertility treatments like intrauterine insemination (IUI), intracervical (at-home) insemination, or in vitro fertilization (IVF). This option supports a wide range of family-building journeys, including those with genetic concerns, same-sex female couples, single women seeking parenthood, and those navigating male infertility.

Whether you're planning to use donor sperm for at-home insemination, IUI, or IVF, your first step is to consult with your preferred healthcare provider. Together, you can create a foundation for your journey.

If you are an eligible recipient for donor sperm, your next step is to find a sperm donor. You have the option to choose someone that you know (a directed donor) or someone you do not know prior to donation (an anonymous donor, who may be open-ID or non-contact) to be your sperm donor.

Sperm Donation—the Donors

Men (assigned males at birth) choose to become sperm donors for various reasons:

- **Altruism**. Some men learn that there is a need for sperm donors and choose to help based on that alone.
- **Personal connection**. This may include being donor-conceived (the sperm donor was conceived with donor sperm or eggs), having friends or family who experienced infertility, or being members of the LGBTQIA+ community.
- **Financial support**. Compensation may help sperm donors pay for college or living expenses, support themselves, or save money for long-term financial goals.

Most commonly, donors say they are donating for a combination of reasons. Some sperm banks will include this information in each donor's profile so you can review your chosen donor's motivation for joining his program.

Once a potential donor finds a program that he would like to join, he must complete an application process, which can take several weeks and involves medical testing, screening, and counseling. This process may vary by program.

The first step in the application process is a semen analysis, which is where most potential sperm donors are disqualified. This important step determines if the potential donor's sperm will be effective in fertility treatments. Certain criteria involved in a semen analysis are the sperm concentration, motility, and morphology (appearance).

If approved, the potential donor will provide detailed health information about himself and his family, including parents, siblings, grandparents, and any children.

Sperm banks should also run background checks and verify records (college degrees, etc.) for each potential donor. Once approved, they will then undergo a mental health assessment and counseling to discuss:

- The long-term implications of donation
- Emotional and ethical considerations
- Future impact on donor-conceived children

Lastly, potential donors must complete medical testing and screening. In the United States, the FDA requires that each potential donor completes infectious disease screening (hepatitis, HIV, etc.) and testing for conditions that could impact future pregnancies and donor-conceived offspring. Some sperm banks may also require extended genetic carrier screening, which determines whether or not a potential donor carries a mutation in one or more of his genes that could be passed on to any donor-conceived offspring.

After all of these steps are completed and everything is reviewed and approved, the donor will actively donate for approximately six to twelve months. The samples are frozen and stored in liquid nitrogen. Donor samples are quarantined for six months while the donor is routinely tested for infectious diseases because some infectious diseases (such as HIV) may not show up in the blood for six months. The FDA also requires that licensed sperm banks perform ongoing infectious disease testing on each donor.

After exiting the program, the donor must update his sperm bank with any relevant health changes that could affect any donor-conceived offspring.

The Safety of Sperm Banks

Though it may seem simpler to bypass a clinic or sperm bank when using donor sperm, it is important to utilize these options because there are protections in place to ensure that you are receiving a safe, viable, and responsibly sourced sample. Clinics and sperm banks offer critical medical, legal, and ethical safeguards that help protect recipients, donors, and future children. Additionally, most clinics and sperm banks require the following:

- **Semen analysis.** Clinics or sperm banks require semen analyses to be completed prior to donor insemination. Semen analyses ensure that the donor's sperm sample is adequate enough to achieve fertilization. For example, you may not want to use sperm from a donor with a very low sperm count or motility since these factors decrease your chances of success.

- **Infectious disease testing.** Health screenings and testing ensure that you are receiving samples that are safe for use. In the United States, the FDA requires that potential sperm donors are screened for infectious diseases such as hepatitis B and C, HIV, and syphilis before they are eligible to become donors. Further, their sperm samples are quarantined for six months, after which time the donor is retested for these diseases since it can take six months for some infections to be detected in the blood. This ensures that the semen samples are completely free of any infectious diseases. If you are seeking treatment in a clinic, you will likely be required to use a donor that completed all required FDA testing and quarantining.

- **Genetic carrier screening**. Most sperm donors are screened for a panel of genetic conditions that they could potentially pass on to any offspring created with their sperm. This is especially important if the egg source (yourself, your partner, or an egg donor) is also a carrier of any genetic conditions. Understanding both sides of the genetic equation helps reduce the risk of inherited disorders. (see Chapter 8).

If you choose to use donor sperm that has not undergone proper testing and screening, there is a risk that the sperm might carry infectious diseases or genetic mutations that can be passed on to any offspring created with the sperm. Additionally, you will not know if there is viable sperm present in the sample if a semen analysis is not performed.

It's also important to consider the legal aspects of donor insemination. Clinics and sperm banks require sperm donors and recipients to sign consents that clarify parental rights and responsibilities, protect donor-conceived children, and establish legal boundaries and protections for all parties. If you're considering donor sperm outside of a regulated clinic or bank, it's strongly recommended that you consult with an attorney who specializes in third-party reproduction. Legal guidance ensures that everyone's rights are protected.

Choosing and Receiving Donor Sperm

1. **Choosing a donor.** It's important to begin your search for a sperm donor early so you have ample time to browse the available donors from multiple sperm banks and consider what factors are most important for your family-building goals. This is a very important decision, so do not feel rushed to choose your donor. Most sperm banks offer limited donor profile information for free. Take advantage of this information and use it to narrow down your choices before purchasing access to more detailed information about these donors. Also, keep in mind that there are multiple levels of access available (the cost increases with each level), so make sure that you are getting the right amount of important information about each donor.

Basic profile details may include:

- Ethnicity
- Hair and eye color
- Height and weight
- Education and profession
- Genetic carrier results and CMV (cytomegalovirus) status
- Generalized impressions of the donor's personality and physical traits

Expanded profiles may include:

- Photos or childhood images
- Audio interviews or written statements from the donor
- Details about physical characteristics such as left/right-handed, birth weight, and hair texture
- Personal and family health information
- More in-depth information about personality, such as hobbies, interests, and personality insights

2. **Purchasing vials.** Donor vials can sell out quickly, so be prepared to purchase *multiple* vials before you begin fertility treatment. If your preferred donor has limited vials available, your sperm bank can provide waitlist information or insights into when more vials are being released.

Different sperm banks may offer multiple vial options that vary based on their sperm concentrations and whether or not the sample has been washed. The washing process removes other components of the semen, leaving only sperm cells in the final sample, while unwashed samples contain all of the contents of the ejaculate (see Chapter 7). Fertility clinics should be able to use either type of vial because they have the ability to wash the samples before use. If you are pursuing at-home insemination, you can also use either type of vial because the sperm cells will naturally separate from the other contents of the semen and swim into the uterus. The most common vial type is the washed vial, which can be used for any clinical or at-home treatment. If you are using a special type of vial, or if this is the only vial left from your chosen donor, talk with your healthcare provider ahead of time because he/she may prefer that you have higher sperm counts or require multiple vials to optimize your chances of success.

Since many fertility clinics charge fees to store donor sperm, many sperm banks provide storage options with your vial purchase. Be sure to check out what is included with your vial purchase to find out if you have free storage options with your treatment.

3. **Shipping vials.** Early shipping ensures that your vials are ready when you need them Here are some tips for a smooth delivery:

- Coordinate a shipment with your sperm bank to ensure that your vials will be at your home or fertility clinic at least three days before your fertility treatment.
- If you have storage options at your clinic, consider shipping your vials sooner if you do not have to pay a storage fee.
- For home insemination, ask if your sperm bank offers larger shipping tanks that will keep your vials frozen until you are ready to use them.

Considerations for the Use of Donor Sperm

Whether you are choosing to use a directed or anonymous donor, there are some important questions to ask yourself when planning your treatment with donor sperm, including:

- Do you plan on having more than one child? Would you like all of your children to be conceived with sperm from the same donor?
- If you are in a same-sex relationship, do you and/or a partner both plan to carry pregnancies?
- Is giving your children the option of future contact with their donor (if open-ID) important?

- Do you have any genetic conditions that should be considered when choosing a donor?
- Would you like to connect with other families who used the same donor?
- Is the number of families who use your donor important? (Banks have various limits when it comes to family size. On the other hand, your directed donor may only donate to you.)

If you have access to a counselor who specializes in donor conception (either through your fertility clinic or someone local or online), consider speaking with them to discuss these questions and more. They can help you explore your values, clarify your goals, and feel confident when choosing a sperm donor that fits your needs.

Haley's Story

I always knew I wanted to be a mother and had planned to do it alone for as long as I can remember. I started my career, bought a house, traveled, and really enjoyed my life until I felt ready to start my fertility journey.

At age thirty, I went to a local fertility clinic to test my reproductive health. I was diagnosed with lean PCOS and a low ovarian reserve. This was sad and rather shocking news because I was young and very healthy, which I thought would be enough to conceive. My doctor advised me that, if I was planning to become a mother, I should start as soon as possible.

My journey started with an IUI procedure, which involved the interesting and overwhelming process of choosing a donor's sperm. There were many factors to consider in my decision, such as each donor's type of identification disclosure, hair and skin color, and genetic issues. Once I selected a donor, the donor sperm was shipped to my clinic and I started the cycle. There were countless appointments, pills, and injections leading up to the procedure. It sometimes felt very lonely doing all of these things alone, but the end hope of becoming a mother kept me moving forward.

My first IUI failed and so did my second. This was a huge gut punch to me. I lost my excitement about the process and became rather apathetic to the whole thing. My next decision was to go through another IUI or move forward with an egg retrieval and IVF cycle. I decided to go with IVF because, although it was way more costly, it would hopefully preserve my fertility (since my ovarian reserve was already low) and give me a higher chance of having a live birth.

> *At the end of my IVF cycle, I ended up with five frozen "embabies." I am currently going through a frozen embryo transfer cycle and am very excited to have my first transfer to hopefully become a Mom!*
>
> *This process has been extremely difficult, lonely, tiring, and mentally and physically painful. To help, I have shared with my parents and close friends, who have all been unbelievably supportive throughout my journey. They listen to me, ask lots of questions, and have been there to help with rides, injections, and whatever else I may need.*
>
> *All of that said, this has been worth it! Knowing that I can go through something as difficult and invasive as fertility treatment shows me that I can handle anything going forward. I am thrilled to have multiple chances to become a Mom and hopefully be one of the success stories.*
>
> *My story isn't the norm. I hope that my story empowers single women to know that they have options if they want children. And I hope it shows them that they can do it as single parents and that there are many types of support other than a partner. And finally, I hope it encourages women to get their reproductive health tested, especially because age is working against all of us.*

Donor Oocyte (Egg) Information

The information in this section was contributed by Theresa Færch, managing director US, Cryos International.

Egg donation is a process where a woman (the donor) has eggs retrieved from her ovaries and relinquishes the ownership rights to those eggs and any embryos that are created from them. The intended parent(s) then obtain ownership of some or all of the donated eggs for use in IVF.

There are many reasons why a person or couple might pursue donor eggs as part of their fertility journey, including:

- Fertility issues that prevent a woman from getting pregnant using her own eggs. A common fertility issue is diminished ovarian reserve (DOR), meaning that there are a reduced number of good-quality eggs remaining in the ovaries. This can result in a low number of eggs retrieved, poor fertilization, abnormal embryo development, failed implantation, and/or miscarriage.

- Loss of ovarian function, often due to medical conditions such as cancer or its treatments.
- Absence of ovaries, either congenital or following surgical removal.
- Multiple failed IVF cycles using a woman's own eggs.
- Risk of passing on a genetic condition to offspring.
- Same-sex male couples or single males who cannot biologically produce eggs.
- Other personal or medical reasons.

Some IVF clinics offer on-site egg donation programs, but typically donor eggs are created and stored at donor eggs banks. When a recipient selects and purchases a cohort of donor eggs, they are shipped to the clinic where IVF will be performed.

Reasons to Become an Egg Donor

Surveys have found that the primary reason people donate their eggs is altruism, or the desire to help another person or couple build their families. In many situations, donors have had a friend or family member who has needed to use donor eggs, which motivates them to become donors. The other most common reason is the financial incentive of egg donation since donors are compensated for their time, travel, and medical procedures.

The Egg Donation Process

1. Application. Most large egg banks begin with an online application. Applicants are screened for general health factors such as age, BMI, and smoking status. In some programs, the initial application is more involved and asks for information such as one's family, psychological, and reproductive histories. In other programs, a full application is only completed if the initial application is accepted.
2. Screening and testing. Once these applications are accepted, potential donors undergo rigorous testing and screening, which may involve a physical and pelvic exam, blood work, infectious disease screening, background check, genetic screening, and mental health evaluation. In the United States, the FDA requires specific screening to be performed

on each donor before she can donate her eggs. Some donors will also be asked to submit additional information for their donor profiles, such as baby photos and a list of their hobbies, which will be used to match their donated eggs with a recipient(s).

3. Ovarian stimulation and egg retrieval. Once cleared, donors begin ovarian stimulation to produce multiple eggs. After retrieval, the donor relinquishes all rights to the eggs and any resulting embryos.

This entire process typically takes two to four months.

Egg Donation Ineligibility

Fewer than 2 percent of applicants are accepted into a program. Common causes of disqualification include having a(n):

- Infectious disease(s)
- High BMI
- Medical condition (self or family) that can pose a risk to offspring
- Genetic condition that can be passed onto offspring
- Low ovarian reserve (a low number of eggs) or poor egg quality

What is the Process for Receiving Donor Eggs from an Egg Bank?

1. **Choose an egg bank.** Select a bank based on your fertility specialist's recommendations and your personal priorities. Consider factors like donor screening protocols, the diversity of the donor pool, success rates, transparency in pricing, and available support services. You will need to register with this egg bank and complete all necessary paperwork and requirements, which can vary between egg banks.

2. **Select a donor.** Once affiliated with an egg bank, you'll gain access to their donor database. Most donor egg banks or in-house programs have online catalogs where you can browse all of its available donors' profiles and select the donor who most appeals to you. This is an important decision that can feel overwhelming at times. Do not rush to

make this decision, and explore all of your options before making a final decision.

3. **Ship the eggs.** If applicable, the donor eggs should be shipped to your fertility clinic *a few weeks before your IVF cycle begins*. The shipment process is coordinated between your fertility clinic and egg bank. Eggs are typically shipped overnight in a shipping tank that is designed to keep them frozen throughout the shipment process. Once the eggs arrive at your IVF clinic, they are safely transferred to and stored in a liquid nitrogen storage tank.

4. **Inseminate the eggs.** On the day of insemination, the eggs are thawed (unless you are using fresh that are retrieved on the same day as insemination) and placed into culture medium (fluid) in an incubator. Thawed eggs must be fertilized through intracytoplasmic sperm injection (ICSI). The remainder of the IVF cycle then completed in the IVF lab (see Chapter 7).

Splitting Up Eggs from a Single Donor

On average, fifteen to twenty eggs are retrieved from each egg donor. Many donor egg banks/programs divide these eggs into lots of six to eight eggs. However, some donor egg banks/programs allow recipients to own all of the eggs from a single retrieval. It's also possible for a recipient to purchase multiple lots of the same donor's eggs, and there is no limit to the number of eggs that can be received. However, many egg banks/clinics allow lots of a donor's eggs to be received by multiple people/couples. Talk with your egg bank/program about lot sizes, exclusivity, and availability before selecting a donor.

Egg Donor Identification

An egg donor's identity can be known (directed donation) or unknown (anonymous or nonidentified). Alternatively, open-ID donation is when the donor agrees to be contacted by the donor-conceived child once the child reaches legal age (usually eighteen). Advances in genetic testing and online databases mean anonymity may not be guaranteed long-term.

So, why even offer anonymous egg donation? Some countries only allow anonymous egg donors, and some individuals/couples do not plan to disclose to their offspring that they were donor conceived. Donors and recipients should be counseled about the potential for children created through donor eggs to ultimately discover the identities of their egg donors later in life.

In some situations, recipients know the identities of their egg donors before the eggs are donated. An example of this situation would be if a friend of the parent(s) agreed to donate her eggs to the parent(s). This process is typically completed through a fertility clinic and has the same requirements mentioned above.

Other Considerations

1. **Do your research**. Don't settle on one donor egg bank/program until you've explored your options. This is a step-by-step process that can take time, it's very important and should not be rushed .

2. **Use your resources**. Fertility counselors, donor coordinators, and legal professionals can guide you through each step of the egg donation or reception process.

3. **Don't get discouraged**. Though many potential egg donors are not able to donate their eggs, do not get discouraged by this low number if you are considering donating your eggs. It costs nothing to apply to become an egg donor, and you have the amazing opportunity to help another person or couple create a family. If you are searching for a donor, remember that there are many donors available through different donor egg banks/programs, so do not get discouraged if you do not immediately find a donor that appeals to you.

Barbara's Story

Over seven years ago, I was diagnosed with low ovarian reserve (a low number of eggs in my ovaries) on top of my already-existing endometriosis and massive fibroids. Our doctor informed us that I could not use my own eggs for IVF, so our options were adoption or egg donation.

We went the adoption route and, four long years later, were still in the waiting process. So, we decided to try egg donation. We reached out to an egg bank and they showed us a database of their egg donors. It was rather surreal for us to choose an egg donor from a place that looked kind of like a dating website.

> *We ended up choosing a lovely lady whose personality was a good fit for us. We then met her online and chatted with her for almost an hour. She was very friendly, and we knew she was the right fit for us.*
>
> *It can be very difficult to consider egg donation and choose an egg donor. I knew that I wanted children from an early age, so it didn't matter to me if my child was genetically linked to me. I knew I would love that child regardless.*
>
> *I think that by sharing about egg donation it can really help other couples who might not know about egg donation or might be on the fence about it. It's an amazing other way to have a child and there is no reason to hide it. Shining a light on egg donation and known egg donation is so important!*

Embryo Donation and Adoption

The information in this section was contributed by Elizabeth Button, executive director of the Snowflakes Embryo Adoption Program.

If a person or couple has additional embryos frozen at a fertility clinic that they do not wish to discard or donate to research, they have the option to donate these embryos to another couple or person for reproductive use. In turn, these embryos can be adopted by recipients who hope to use the embryos to build their families. In the United States, embryos are governed by property law, and each program will manage legal contracts differently. In general, these contracts transfer ownership of embryos from the donating person or couple to the adopting person or couple. Policies vary by country, and some regions have stricter regulations around fertility treatment and embryo donation.

Embryo Donation Process

Each program has its own requirements and procedures for donating embryos. It's important to understand your program's policies before pursuing embryo donation.

In the United States, embryo donors must complete FDA-required infectious disease testing (e.g., HIV, hepatitis B and C) before they qualify to donate their embryos to another person. If a donor tests positive for certain infectious diseases, the embryos may not be eligible for adoption through some programs or clinics.

Though it is not currently required by the FDA, some IVF clinics also request that embryo donors undergo genetic carrier screening, which determines if the egg and/or sperm provider carries any genetic mutations that can be passed on to the embryos that they created together.

If donor eggs and/or sperm were used to create the embryos, the contract with the sperm or egg providers must be reviewed to ensure that the embryo donors have permission to donate their remaining embryos to another person or couple.

Most programs collect a minimal amount of information regarding the medical history of the egg and sperm providers for potential embryo recipients to review. Some programs also require more in-depth medical histories of the sperm and egg providers that often contain information dating back two or more generations. If donor eggs or sperm were utilized to create the embryos, medical history may be limited.

Matching between donors and recipients is often done online through self-matching platforms or by agency staff. Keep in mind that some programs prioritize donor preferences, while others prioritize recipient needs. It's important to research the specifics of any program to see if the matching process aligns with your personal expectations.

Key Information About Donated Embryos

The fertility clinics that recipients intend to use for their frozen embryo transfers will usually require the following information about the adopted embryos:

- The year they were created and frozen
- Their developmental stage and grade prior to being frozen
- How they were frozen (slow freezing versus vitrification)
- Preimplantation genetic testing results, if available
- The type of device they are frozen on and the number of embryos per device

Known Versus Anonymous Donations

An anonymous donation means that neither the donor nor the recipient receives identifying information about one another. In these situations, no communication is facilitated nor established. This includes information about how many people received embryos from the same donors, along with information regarding genetic siblings. Realistically, anonymous donation is not always a possibility in the world today due to the invention of DNA test kits, social media, and online registries.

In a known match, the adopting and receiving parties mutually agree upon the level of communication they wish to have at the time of adoption. Relationships may evolve over time, and many programs offer tools to help facilitate communication while everyone gets to know each other.

Splitting Up Donated Embryos

Some programs will divide embryo sets, also referred to as cohorts (embryos from the same donor), among multiple recipients due to the high demand for donated embryos. In these situations, receiving parents will only receive one or two embryos, and neither the donor nor the recipients are given information about the distribution of the genetic sibling embryos. Therefore, there is often no tracking or permanent record of genetic siblings born into multiple families. If a program only allows the recipient one to two embryos per embryo transfer and the transfer is unsuccessful, the recipient may need to pay additional fees for future matches.

Other programs will place all of a donor's embryos with one recipient. This can allow the recipient's family to have multiple genetic siblings and multiple frozen embryo transfers without having to return to the program to be matched with additional embryos.

Reasons to Adopt Embryos

Many people who decide to use donated embryos have been diagnosed with female, male, or unexplained infertility and have completed multiple unsuccessful IVF cycles with or without donor gametes (eggs and sperm). Others may simply be interested in giving donated embryos a chance to be born. In some cases, medical or personal circumstances make embryo adoption the best path forward.

Embryo Adoption Process

As with embryo donation, the process for adopting embryos may vary between programs or agencies. Adopters should complete their own research regarding the programs that are available, including:

- Researching and contacting programs that align with their expectations
- Choosing between self-matching versus agency support
- Ensuring that the clinic or program has embryos available
- Determining what sort of relationship is desired with the donor

Adopting families may also need to complete other administrative documentation before officially being accepted into a program, which may include a family evaluation or home study.

After families are matched, legal contracts are signed and the adopted embryos are shipped (if applicable) to the adopting family's fertility clinic. Once the embryos arrive at the adopting family's clinic, a frozen embryo transfer (FET) can be planned and scheduled. On the day of the scheduled embryo transfer, an embryo is thawed and transferred into the uterus of the intended mother or gestational carrier. In most cases, only one embryo is transferred at a time.

Embryo Adoption Ineligibility

The requirements to adopt embryos may differ between programs. The primary reason that someone may not be able to adopt embryos is that their fertility specialist may determine that they are not able to carry a pregnancy to term. In these situations, many families use a gestational carrier to carry a pregnancy to term. Additional reasons are that the adopting family may not be approved to adopt include significant criminal history, or age restrictions based on program criteria.

J and J's Story

My husband and I have been TTC for nearly six years. All of our labs appeared normal and no superficial issues were seen aside from stage 3 endometriosis, but our real issue came down to egg quality.

> After three egg retrievals, I was never able to make a viable embryo. When my cousin offered to donate her eggs to us, we went for it. After she underwent two egg retrievals, we ended up with five day 3 embryos. Unfortunately, our first transfer resulted in a miscarriage and the following three transfers failed.
>
> While preparing to end our fertility journey, we stumbled across embryo donation. Not only was it far more affordable than using donor eggs, but we were able to privately match and develop a relationship with a donor. This means that our potential children will have answers to any questions they may have in their futures!
>
> Donor conception is not widely spoken about, but my husband and I would likely never have a family without it. I wanted to experience a pregnancy, and our donor's family members wanted to give another family a chance to give life to their embryos. Our story is going to be different from many families, but it is a story of love.
>
> I hope that my story informs families of other options that aren't well known, including embryo adoption. Donor conception can be a beautiful way to grow your family.

Surrogacy

The information in this section was contributed by Dawn Baker, CEO of US Surrogacy, LLC.

Surrogacy offers a powerful and affirming way to build a family when carrying a pregnancy isn't possible or advisable. Gestational surrogacy involves a gestational carrier (surrogate) who carries a pregnancy to term for another person or family. This differs from traditional surrogacy, in which the surrogate uses her own eggs and is biologically related to the child. Gestational surrogacy is the most common and legally supported form of surrogacy in the United States. It requires IVF, during which the intended parent's or a donor's eggs are fertilized in an IVF lab with the intended parent's or a donor's sperm. A resulting embryo is transferred into the uterus of the surrogate in an attempt to initiate a pregnancy. Therefore, the surrogate is not biologically related to the baby.

Surrogates may be known to the intended parents (e.g., a friend or relative) or matched through a surrogacy agency. The level of involvement between a surrogate and intended parents varies and should be discussed early in the process.

When to Consider Surrogacy

In some situations, people or couples know that they will require a surrogate before they begin fertility treatment. Examples include same-sex male couples, single males, or women with certain medical conditions that prevent them from carrying a pregnancy.

Others arrive at surrogacy after multiple failed IVF cycles or when advised by their fertility specialist that carrying a pregnancy is no longer safe or feasible. If you're emotionally and physically exhausted from repeated failed embryo transfers, surrogacy may offer a renewed path forward.

Becoming a Surrogate

Most women choose to become surrogates through agencies, as they help navigate the complex process. The potential surrogate completes an application process, which often includes a medical and psychological screening, before being admitted into the agency's program. Once accepted, the surrogate will likely complete additional testing and screening, including a background check. She then enters the matching process, which might involve screening profiles or meeting (virtual or in-person) with prospective intended parents. Once a match has been made and legal contracts have been signed, the surrogate will complete additional testing and may also complete procedures (e.g., a saline sonohysterogram to evaluate her uterus) prior to the transfer. The embryo transfer can then be scheduled following the instructions provided by the fertility clinic that will perform the embryo transfer. If the transfer is successful, the surrogate will attend routine prenatal appointments and ultrasounds throughout the pregnancy.

Choosing a Surrogate

While some people pursue independent surrogacy (no agency is involved), many intended parents work with agencies. Each agency may have unique requirements, so it's best to talk with various agencies about their process during an initial consultation. In many agencies, the intended parent(s) will complete an application and, if approved, may complete a psychological and/or medical screening and background check. The intended parent(s) can then begin the matching process, which might involve screening profiles and meeting (virtual or in-person) with potential surrogates. Once a match has been made and legal contracts have been signed, the intended parent(s) and surrogate will work together throughout the pregnancy until the baby is delivered.

Coping with Surrogacy

Emotionally, surrogacy can be bittersweet. Some intended parents feel relief and hope, while others experience varying levels of grief, guilt, or sadness. This is especially true if they have envisioned themselves carrying their own child. Letting go of that vision can be painful, but it's also a step toward healing and embracing a new path to parenthood. All emotions surrounding surrogacy are valid, and fertility counselors can help you process your emotions and find peace.

Other Considerations

If you are considering surrogacy, you may want to consider the following:

- Start the process early. Waitlists for qualified surrogates can be long—sometimes six months to several years. The sooner you get on a waitlist, the sooner you'll have options and surrogate candidates to consider.
- When meeting with surrogacy agencies for the first time, make sure you've done your research before the consultation and come prepared with questions.
- Avoid putting down a nonrefundable deposit with a surrogacy agency before being matched. Unfortunately, surrogacy scams do exist, and there have been intended parents who've lost nonrefundable deposits and never matched with a qualified surrogate.
- Before you match with your surrogate, think about the type of relationship you want to have with her. Do you envision a close friendship with regular communication, or do you prefer to have more boundaries and less connection? There's no right or wrong answer, and a skilled surrogacy agency owner will be able to find you a match that reflects your needs.
- When it comes to matching with your surrogate, stay flexible on your criteria. Surrogates are real-life people, and they are not perfect human beings. Focus on whether they can safely carry your child when making your choice.

Surrogacy may not be part of your original plan, but it has helped thousands of families grow for many years. Talk with your fertility specialist if you are considering surrogacy as part of your treatment.

A Surrogate's Letter to Intended Parents

As a woman and a mother, I understand the deeply rooted desire within us to become parents and have our own children, and I deeply sympathize with those who need medical intervention to build their family and welcome a baby.

I know that surrogacy is almost never the first choice for intended parents, especially for those who've undergone IVF treatments without success. It takes so much trust and courage to open yourself up to the possibility of having a baby through surrogacy, and this process is usually not done overnight. It takes deep reflection to come to a place where you're ready to consider working with a surrogate.

We refer to surrogacy as a "journey" because it truly is a road that winds and twists with a destination unknown. Not unlike IVF itself, surrogacy can be filled with moments ranging from the happiest highs, to the unexpected lows, and quite honestly a lot of waiting in between. .

As a surrogate myself, I wanted to give some perspective to Intended Parents on why I decided to become a surrogate. I had the rare advantage of working in the surrogacy industry for years before my own surrogacy journey began, and I was able to witness firsthand the pure joy that surrogacy gives to parents. Being able to see those who have endured countless miscarriages and failed transfers finally being able to hold their baby in their arms is just an overwhelming emotion that moves you to your core. In that moment, all the struggle is forgotten and she is the mother she was always meant to be.

When Intended Parents are looking into the process of surrogacy, it is fair to be wary or concerned about the motivation of a surrogate candidate. And I will not deny that the compensation for surrogates can be a motivating factor. But I can attest to the fact that most surrogates feel the same way I do. We are mothers who love our children deep in our souls, and we are in a place where we can help others find their own unconditional love. Once your own heart is so full, it just feels like the natural step to pass on your good fortune to others.

I hope these words can put anyone considering surrogacy a little more at ease, and maybe even provide that little push to make the first step. It's a long road ahead, but it's the most rewarding treasure at the end of the journey.

—*Gennifer Rose*

Surrogate and Founder of SurrogacyMama.com

Adoption: A Guide to Domestic Infant Adoption

Submitted by Amy Twombly & Caitlin Phillips, LCSW, Co-Founders and Executive Partners of Hello Baby Adoption Consultants.

Adoption is a profound, life-changing process that reshapes the lives of both children and families. As defined by the Child Welfare Information Gateway, "Adoption is the social, emotional, and legal process in which children who will not be raised by their birth parents become full and permanent legal members of another family while maintaining genetic and psychological connections to their birth family."

There are three primary types of adoption:

1. **Domestic Infant Adoption**
2. **Foster-to-Adopt**
3. **International Adoption**

This section focuses on domestic infant adoption, where an expectant mother chooses to place her child with an adoptive family, typically at birth.

Paths to Domestic Infant Adoption

Adoptive families can pursue adoption through several avenues, each of which offers different levels of support, legal oversight, and matching services. Common examples are:

- **Self-matching** (finding an expectant mother independently)
- **Working with an adoption attorney**
- **Signing on with a licensed adoption agency**
- **Engaging an adoption consultant**

Levels of Openness in Adoption

Adoption can vary in terms of openness. The level of contact between adoptive families and birth parents, categorized as follows:

- **Open adoption**: The birth mother selects and maintains direct contact with the adoptive family (e.g., visits, calls).
- **Semi-open**: The birth mother selects the adoptive family, and communication after placement is mediated through an agency. This often involves the exchange of pictures and letters.
- **Closed adoption**: There is no contact between the birth and adoptive families before or after placement. In some cases, the birth mother may not choose the adoptive family.

The Domestic Infant Adoption Process

The domestic infant adoption process can generally be broken down into four phases:

Phase One: Preparing for Adoption

An adoptive family completes a home study, which assesses their suitability to provide a loving, stable, and secure home for a child. This study is conducted by a licensed agency or an independent provider. Additionally, the family creates a profile book (typically a mix of photos and text) to introduce themselves to expectant mothers. Families can create their own or use a professional profile designer.

Phase Two: Waiting Family

Adoptive families may work with agencies or attorneys, depending on state regulations, to find adoption opportunities. Each state has unique adoption laws, and the requirements for adoptive families vary. Families become "waiting families" once they are approved and ready to present their profile book to expectant mothers for consideration. When chosen, families enter a "match" with the expectant mother, formalized through a contract and fee.

Phase Three: Match and Placement

Once a match is established, the adoptive family and expectant mother may begin building a relationship while awaiting the baby's arrival. The relationship is typically facilitated by a social worker. If the expectant mother wishes, the adoptive family may attend the hospital for the birth of the baby. The level of involvement will be based on the expectant mother's desires for labor, delivery, and postpartum.

If the birth mother proceeds with the adoption plan after the birth of the baby, she signs relinquishment consents according to state law, and the baby is placed with the adoptive family. The agency assumes legal rights of the baby and allows the adoptive family "placement" of the baby with the goal of permanent adoption. Out-of-state families must await ICPC (Interstate Compact on the Placement of Children) clearance before returning home.

Phase Four: Post-Placement and Finalization

Once home, the adoptive family will begin a post-placement period before they are able to legally finalize the adoption. The post-placement period involves supervised visits by the social worker who completed the family's home study. Once this period concludes, the adoption is finalized in court, and the family is granted full legal rights. The process typically takes about three to six months, depending on state regulations. The post-placement period ensures the adoption is in the child's best interest and that the adoptive family is comfortable with the permanent placement.

Emotional Aspects of Adoption

Adoption is often described as an emotional rollercoaster. Common feelings include:

- **Fear**: Concerns about bonding with a non-biological child, financial stress, or whether the birth mother will change her mind.
- **Excitement**: Joy when presenting a profile book, being chosen, attending the birth, and finalizing the adoption.
- **Anxiety**: Worries about making the right decisions and whether they will ever be selected.

- **Disappointment**: The sadness of not being chosen or if a birth mother decides to parent her child.
- **Happiness**: Celebrating milestones and welcoming a child into your family.

Families are encouraged to process any unresolved grief, particularly surrounding infertility, before embarking on the adoption journey. Counseling and support groups are valuable resources throughout this process.

Benefits and Challenges of Domestic Infant Adoption

Benefits

- Adoption offers families the chance to grow and fulfill their dreams of parenting.
- Adoption offers a baby a stable, caring environment, often with families eager to provide the emotional, financial, and physical resources the child needs to thrive.
- Open adoptions, which are increasingly common, allow adoptive families to maintain a relationship with the birth family. This can benefit the child by providing a sense of identity and connection to their roots. It also allows adoptive families to have ongoing communication, which can contribute to the child's emotional well-being.
- Adopting a child connects families to a larger, supportive community made up of adoptees, birth parents, and other adoptive families. This network provides shared experiences, advice, and understanding, offering valuable emotional support throughout the adoptive family's journey.

These benefits contribute to fulfilling, positive experiences for adoptive families, birth parents, and adoptees alike, fostering lifelong connections and creating loving, supportive environments for the child.

Challenges

- Adoption is expensive and typically self-funded, making it difficult for families to afford.
- Expectant mothers choosing adoption are not always in the best of circumstances, which is why they might be pursuing adoption for their child. For example, they may have mental health struggles, abuse illegal substances, or be in an overall difficult situation.
- Adoption is not a 100 percent guarantee. Birth mothers have a period of time before they relinquish their rights. During this time, the birth mother can decide that she wants to parent and not move forward with adoption. If a birth mother chooses to parent, the adoptive family typically loses nonrefundable fees.
- Adoption involves a triad of people: birth parents, adoptees, and adoptive parents. Often, there is a relationship among all members of the adoption triad in an open adoption. Navigating these lifelong relationships can be both wonderful and challenging, but adoptive families must realize that these relationships are often in the best interest of the child.

Adoptive families should prepare for these challenges through education, support, and realistic expectations about the process and relationships involved. The more prepared and educated families are, the smoother the process will be.

Adoptive families should strive to understand the emotions and circumstances of birth parents while always centering the child's well-being.

Key Considerations Before Starting the Adoption Journey

Adoptive families should connect with trusted adoption professionals who will guide them through each step of the process. These may include home study providers, adoption consultants, licensed agencies, adoption attorneys, and profile designers. It's essential to read reviews, seek referrals, and check online support groups to find professionals who align with their values and needs.

They should also thoroughly educate themselves on several critical topics:

- **Expectant parent circumstances**: Most expectant mothers considering adoption are in their late 20s or 30s and often have other children. They are typically navigating crisis situations and are not the stereotypical image of a teen parent.

- **Adoption costs**: Costs can be offset by loans, grants, fundraising, employer stipends, and the federal adoption tax credit.
- **Prenatal substance exposure:** It's crucial for adoptive families to understand how exposure to drugs or alcohol in utero can affect a child's development, health, and behavior. This knowledge empowers families to make thoughtful, informed choices.
- **Transracial adoption**: Families adopting across racial lines must be prepared to honor and support their child's cultural identity. This includes ongoing education, community engagement, and intentional representation.
- **Open adoption**: Most birth parents prefer some level of openness, which is beneficial for the child's identity, emotional well-being, and sense of belonging.
- **Timeframe**: The adoption process can take up to twelve months or more, depending on factors such as family preferences, the adoption path, and legal and logistical factors.

Chapter 13
Nurturing Supportive Relationships

The information in this chapter was contributed by Karyn Rosenberg, LCSW, PMH-C.

Supporting someone experiencing infertility or pregnancy loss is both an act of love and emotional courage. While it's natural to want to help, finding the right words and actions can be challenging. This chapter offers guidance on how to show up with empathy, sensitivity, and respect while recognizing that each person's experience is unique and may evolve over time. Keep in mind that the advice in this chapter might not apply to everyone who is experiencing infertility or loss, especially in severe circumstances.

What Doesn't Help

Infertility and pregnancy loss are often accompanied by grief, frustration, anger, hopelessness, isolation, and emotional exhaustion. Well-meaning comments and gestures can unintentionally cause harm, so be mindful of your words and actions while offering support.

Here are some things to avoid:

- **Don't minimize their feelings.** Statements such as:
  - "Just relax, it'll happen."
  - "You're worrying too much. It will happen when it's meant to happen."
  - "You're still young. You have time to have a baby. It's not a big deal."

  can dismiss the immense pain and sorrow they may be experiencing. This can be particularly hurtful as it implies that their situation isn't serious, which can make them feel invalidated and alone. These comments may also imply that their infertility is a matter of mindset, not a complex medical issue. Infertility can be a life crisis for those affected and should be treated with the seriousness it deserves.

- **Don't ask intrusive questions** such as:
  - "When are you going to have a baby?"
  - "Why are you doing IVF?"
  - "Have you considered adoption?"

  These questions can feel invasive and judgmental, adding pressure to an already vulnerable situation.

- **Don't attribute their infertility to destiny or fate.** Phrases like:
  - "Everything happens for a reason."
  - "This is God's will."

  may feel invalidating and imply they are being punished, which can deepen their emotional distress.

- **Don't give unsolicited advice.** When you suggest all of the things that the person should try in order to get pregnant, such as:
  - Treatment options ("just do IVF")
  - Miracle cures ("my friend tried this and got pregnant right away!")
  - Supplements
  - Diets
  - Other lifestyle changes

  you sound insensitive because you may not know what the person has already tried or from which professionals they are already receiving guidance and/or treatment. These suggestions can feel like blame and may not take into account the complex emotional and financial realities that shape their journey. And keep in mind that just because some miracle solution worked for another person does not mean that it will work for them.

- **Don't assume the treatment worked**. IVF helps a lot of people have children, but it doesn't guarantee success for everyone. Please don't say things like: "how far along are you now?" after an IVF cycle. This can reopen wounds and cause additional stress.
- **Don't compare your experience to theirs**. Phrases like:
  - "I know how you feel, I also tried for a few months
  - Your cousin got pregnant without trying."

  can trivialize their journey and make them feel unseen or unheard.
- **Avoid toxic positivity.** Statements like:
  - "I know it will work this time!"
  - "You'll be pregnant in no time!"

    cause more harm than good. Even though you mean well, these statements exchange genuine empathy and support for superficial encouragement. Toxic positivity dismisses and invalidates the complex struggle that someone is going through.
- **Never say "at least."** When you say things like:
  - "At least you know you can get pregnant" following a miscarriage
  - "At least you can do another round of IVF" after a failed IVF cycle

    it shifts the focus away from their pain and invalidates their grief. This can make them feel unheard and unsupported.
- **Be mindful of your jokes about parenthood.** If you have children, don't say things like:
  - "Take my kids for a day and you'll be glad you don't have any."
  - "If you really want a baby, you can always borrow mine."

    These statements sound cruel as the person very much would like to have a child, and this dismisses their longing for parenthood.

If you have said or done some of these things, try not to worry. It is not too late to be self-aware and make changes. Even small shifts in language and behavior can make a profound difference.

What Does Help

If someone is struggling with infertility, your support will make such a difference in their healing and resilience. Here are meaningful ways to "show up" for a loved one navigating this journey:

- **Offer realistic and practical help.** A simple "What can I do to help?" can go a long way. Whether it's running errands, attending appointments, or dropping off a meal, small gestures show you care. Don't pressure them for an answer—just let them know you're available.
- **Be an attentive listener.** Truly hearing what your loved one is saying and being present is one of the most helpful things you can do. Offer a safe space to talk and listen without judgment, advice, or interruption. Just be there for them, either in the moment or when they need to talk.
- **Validate their feelings**. Remind your loved one that it's okay not to be okay. Acknowledge their pain, frustration, and grief. Let them know you'll be there through the highs and lows.
- **Take time to learn about the process.** Learn about infertility and IVF through books, podcasts, or videos. Your effort to understand their experience shows your commitment and compassion.
- **Encourage self-care.** Support activities that reduce stress, such as meditation, journaling, walks, and massages. Remind them that self-care is not selfish; it's essential.
- **Practice empathy.** Try to put yourself in their shoes. Infertility is unpredictable. Some days may feel hopeful, while others may feel heartbreaking. Be flexible and try not to take certain emotions (e.g., anger, frustration) personally.
- **Be mindful of triggers.** Pregnancy announcements, baby showers, and social media posts can be painful and bring up strong emotions for anyone struggling with infertility or loss. If you're expecting, consider sharing the news privately first to give them space to process. Keep in mind that this news may stir up feelings of jealousy or anger, and be prepared to handle these emotions.

- **Celebrate their wins.** The IVF journey can be full of ups and downs, so if your friend or family member has shared something significant with you, be genuine and authentic. Let them know that they are resilient and you are proud of their strength.
- **Keep inviting them.** You may notice that your loved one chooses to stay home more often than usual. This is probably because they are dealing with a lot of emotions and want to process them in their own way. But it doesn't hurt to keep inviting them out to let them know that you care and want to spend time with them. Try not to take it personally if they keep saying no, and respect their boundaries if they do not want to attend.
- **Respect their boundaries.** Your loved one is going through a lot, and some events may be too much for them to handle at any given time. They need to guard their heart. Recognize their limits and try not to overstep them. If you notice that your loved one is in a situation that pushes their boundaries, help remove them from the situation and be there if they need to talk or cry.
- **Check in gently.** A thoughtful message or call can mean a lot. It's okay to ask how they're doing, but don't push them for details. Let them know you're available when they're ready to talk.
- **Be sensitive on social media.** We live in the twenty-first century where social media dominates our lives. Unfortunately, social media can be a minefield for those struggling with infertility because it often presents a curated highlight reel of pregnancies, births, and perfect families. While these posts are well-intentioned, they can be painful reminders of what someone with infertility may be longing for. If you are pregnant or have children, be mindful about some of the content that you share. It may help to share pregnancy news with them privately before posting it on social media to allow them space to process their emotions.

Conclusions

Supporting someone through infertility isn't about fixing their pain, it's about walking beside them with empathy and care. Your presence, sensitivity, and willingness to learn can help them feel less alone and more understood.

One of the most important things you can do on this earth is to let people know they are not alone. —Shannon L. Alder

Raine's Story

I am a 38-year-old mother of 3 from a previous marriage. My tubes were tied the day after the birth of my third child because I was barely hanging on with the marriage I was in. I eventually had the courage to leave shortly after.

Fast forward and now I have been in a committed relationship for over 5 years. My fiancé and I discussed the possibility of children early on and knew that a tubal reversal was possible. After speaking with our local fertility clinic, I had my tubal reversal in 2020.

Two years passed by trying to conceive through ovulation tracking, and then we tried two rounds of natural IUI (intrauterine insemination) with zero results. In 2023, we started IVF with a different clinic that was an hour away from our home.

Five months and two unsuccessful IVF cycles passed. In both cycles, I was not able to produce any day 5 embryos. We are also in a shared-risk protocol through our clinic and our doctor is instructing us to stop. He is not hopeful supplements or anything will help, so we are currently looking for second opinions and holistic ways to improve what they are assuming is poor egg quality. Our plan is to try again in a few months through our shared-risk program.

I think my biggest take away at this point is that this process can be very isolating. I am the first of my friends and family to do IVF and they often just don't know how to be supportive. For example, they don't ask me questions in fear of upsetting me or they simply don't know what to say to me. I do not think they realize that hearing "I am so sorry" means so much.

I often go without saying anything because I don't like to seek help or support, but I would tell families and friends reading this to reach out more. Bring the coffee or tea. Ask for the lunch date.

The mental aspect of IVF is mind blowing, and I was not prepared by my clinic. It's a very dry and transactional relationship, which makes it harder for someone like me, who doesn't want to ask for help, to say that I am having a hard time with the failures or mood swings. For example, I did not expect the two weeks of birth control to make me feel like a hormonal crazy person. When I mentioned it to my nurse, she laughed and said that "it happens." A heads up would have been nice! In the end, I was not prepared and did not expect the mental toll that this process has taken on me.

Directory of Contributors

Dawn Baker is the owner of US Surrogacy, LLC, and much of her enthusiasm for surrogacy comes from her experience as an infertility patient prior to having her second son and the belief that no matter what walk of life you come from, the inherent desire for a family is in many of us. An ardent supporter of the ability to have a family, she became interested in surrogacy through an acquaintance and soon became an advocate for others to help build their families. With the amazing science of reproductive technology, we are blessed to have the means in our society to realize that desire. She is passionate about the ability to work in an environment whose core existence is the growth of the family.

Elizabeth Button holds a Bachelor of Science in Family Science and has worked in the field of social services for nearly thirty years. She has worked for Nightlight Christian Adoptions in various roles for over twenty years, including the past eight and a half years with the Snowflakes Embryo Adoption program. She has been the Snowflakes executive director since January of 2024. Her hobbies include crafting, reading, and watching her children's sporting events. She is married and has four children, including three biological and one who was adopted, and resides in Kentucky.

Meaghan Doyle, MS, CGC is a certified genetic counselor and the founder of DNAide Genetic Counselling. She obtained her undergraduate degree in Genetics and Psychology from the University of Toronto and her Master of Science in Genetic Counseling from Arcadia University. After being hired as a genetic counselor at a fertility clinic, she recognized how few clinics had genetic counselors on staff to support their patients. She founded DNAide Genetic Counselling to help make fertility genetic counselors be more accessible to patients and clinicians. Doyle has expertise in Preimplantation Genetic Testing, mosaicism and aneuploidy in embryos, and donor conception. She also has a special interest in exploring the genetic causes behind infertility and IVF failure. She is passionate about helping fertility patients by providing them with evidence-based information they can understand and ensuring that they are fully supported to make decisions that will be best for them and their families. Doyle also enjoys educating about fertility genetics on social media @DNAideGC, and shares her experiences working as a fertility genetic counselor on her professional account @MeaghanDoyleGC. Doyle is a member of the Canadian Fertility & Andrology Society (CFAS), American Society for Reproductive Medicine (ASRM) and their Genetic Counseling Professional Group (ASRM GCPG), Canadian Association of Genetic Counsellors (CAGC), Ontario Association of Genetic Counsellors (OAGC), and National Society of Genetic Counselors (NSGC).

Theresa Faerch is the managing director, US for Cryos International. She has worked at Cryos International since 2019 and has more than twenty-five years' experience with international management, sales, e-commerce, and marketing in Europe, the United States, and Asia. Faerch also has experience with cross-border leadership and building high-performance teams. She is well-founded in developing corporate global strategies and has a university degree in International Business Administration & Management. Originally from Denmark, Theresa moved permanently to the United States in 2022.

Catherine Gordon is a reproductive endocrinology and infertility physician practicing at the Fertility Center of Southern California. She specializes in infertility, fertility preservation, third-party family building, and PCOS. She is passionate about personalized care and advocacy and is a proud board member of the Maya's Wings Foundation. Gordon graduated magna cum laude with Departmental Honors from the University of Southern California, then attended medical school at the University of Miami Miller School of Medicine and graduated with Research Distinction. She was honored with induction into the Alpha Omega Alpha (AOA) Medical Honor Society and awarded the Joseph A. DeCenzo Award for Excellence in Obstetrics and Gynecology. She completed residency at the University of California Irvine, where she served as the administrative chief of education and was awarded the Phillip J. DiSaia Society Teaching Award for Excellence. She then completed fellowship training at Brigham and Women's Hospital specializing in Reproductive Endocrinology and Infertility and was awarded the Harvard Medical School Outstanding Teacher of Obstetrics and Gynecology Award. She has now joined the team at Fertility Center of Southern California. Gordon strives to provide evidence-based medicine and herself has contributed to the field through research. She has authored over twenty publications in peer-reviewed journals and three book chapters. Her research is focused on optimizing IVF outcomes and improving oocyte yield for oncofertility patients. She has been awarded the NEFS Ferring Grant and the BWH Expanding the Boundaries Grant in support of her research.

Justin Houman is a urologist and fellowship-trained male reproductive medicine and surgery specialist, whose practice is focused on men's health, including male hormone management, sexual and ejaculatory dysfunction, male fertility, male incontinence, and Peyronie's disease. Houman has published multiple manuscripts on men's health, male fertility, and the health effects of wearable technology. His studies have been published in peer-reviewed journals such as the *Journal of the American Medical Association* and the *Journal of Sexual Medicine*. He has also presented his research at the national and international levels. Houman was born and raised in Orange County, California. He completed a bachelor's degree in Anthropology with a minor in Biomedical Research at the University of California at Los Angeles. He then went on to earn his medical doctorate degree at the University of Rochester School of Medicine. He completed his General Surgery internship and Urology residency at Cedars-Sinai Medical Center. Houman continued his training at UCLA Medical Center, having completed a fellowship in the highly specialized field of male reproductive sedicine and surgery. Houman is a member of the American Urological Association, Sexual Medicine Society of North America, International Society of Sexual Medicine, and Los Angeles Urologic Society.

Phoebe Howells, BSc(Hons), MBBch, MRCOG, has been practicing medicine since 2012, with over ten years of specialized experience in obstetrics and gynecology. Her keen interest in fertility led her to complete a clinical fellowship in reproductive medicine at one of London's top fertility units. Currently, she is a senior trainee at a South London hospital and co-chief medical officer for OVUM, a pioneering reproductive wellness brand. OVUM is distinguished by its evidence-based preconception supplements and fully recyclable early detection pregnancy tests, which include immediate access to guided meditation in the event of an unexpected result. Throughout her career, both in clinical practice and with OVUM, Howells has been committed to educating colleagues, patients, and people on key fertility issues. She has authored numerous articles on reproductive health, shared insights at conferences, and participated in fertility trials for women with adenomyosis.

Cynthia Lim, BA, is the director of marketing at Donor Concierge. Lim has had an extensive marketing career with multinational retail and wellness brands while living in Asia. With her diverse global experience, she is skilled at bridging cultures and takes a practical and holistic approach to overcoming challenges. When Lim decided to embark on the journey of motherhood, she had to face her own fertility issues. While working overseas, she researched donors and clinics in the United States, and pursued her goal to be a parent. She now has a very active four-year-old son, and is pleased to be on the Donor Concierge team to help others achieve their dream of having a child. Cynthia holds a BA in International Relations from the University of British Columbia. She speaks fluent English, Mandarin, and Cantonese. She is a yoga and fitness aficionado and also enjoys travel and foreign language films.

Jennifer McLeland, MD, MBA, is a board-certified OB/GYN with a passion for transforming women's healthcare and empowering women. She is the former owner of a busy private practice; combining her executive leadership skills with her ten-plus years of clinical experience, McLeland is currently the medical director for a comprehensive virtual care platform. McLeland holds a Bachelor of Science in Biology from Marshall University, a medical degree from the Joan C. Edwards School of Medicine at Marshall, and an MBA from the Texas McCombs School of Business. She completed her residency in obstetrics and gynecology at Baylor College of Medicine in Houston. McLeland is an active member of several professional organizations, including the American Medical Association, the American Medical Women's Association, and the American College of Obstetricians and Gynecologists.

Alyse Mencias, MS, completed her Master's in Reproductive Clinical Science from Eastern Virginia Medical School. At the time of writing this, Mencias was clinic relations manager at Seattle Sperm Bank, spending time supporting healthcare professionals' all donor sperm needs. In her current role as an account executive at Posterity Health she continues to support clinic relationships to ensure that patients have access to fertility care.

Amy Twombly and **Caitlin Phillips**, LCSW, are the co-founders and executive partners of Hello Baby Adoption Consultants. Twombly was a hopeful adoptive parent and Phillips was a social worker guiding families through the adoption process when their paths first crossed many years ago. With their two unique perspectives and sets of experiences, their connection grew over time and after a good deal of work, thought, and preparation, Hello Baby was born. Since 2018, they have helped hundreds of families say Hello to their baby.

Chiemi Rajamahendran (AKA Miss.Conception Coach) is a published writer and infertility trauma support specialist. She lends her unique voice and expertise to help people better understand, validate, and process their infertility trauma. She uses her platform to raise awareness about the emotions felt and the reality of mental health issues people experience after treatments like IVF/IUI and grief. Through her unique counseling style she helps people heal their infertility experience. She offers worldwide individual and couples teletherapy.

Karyn Rosenberg, LCSW, PMH-C, is licensed by the state of Florida as a clinical social worker. She holds a Master's Degree in Social Work from the Ohio State University, and a Bachelors Degree in Psychology from the University of Texas. She has a private practice in Boca Raton, Florida, where she provides psychotherapy and hypnotherapy services to children, teens, adults, couples, and families. She is a trauma-trained clinician in EMDR (Eye Movement Desensitization and Reprocessing). Rosenberg has extensive experience in general psychotherapy, but she is most specialized in grief, loss, trauma, and reproductive mental health. She holds a certification in perinatal mental health assisting clients with postpartum depression and anxiety. She works in the field of third-party reproduction, offering consultation, mental health screenings and evaluations, and counseling with egg/sperm/embryo donors, gestational carriers, and Intended Parents. She serves as an expert witness on grief and loss issues. Rosenberg has been an invited speaker at professional conferences and serves as a lecturer and trainer for the community. She is invited to work with schools and workplaces offering crisis counseling and providing critical incident stress debriefing. Rosenberg has extensive experience facilitating bereavement support groups and providing professional training. Rosenberg has been an adjunct professor at Florida Atlantic University where she has taught Grief and Bereavement counseling, Issues in Counseling Women, and Issues in Mental Health Counseling on a graduate and undergraduate level. Her professional membership includes the Florida Society of Oncology Social Workers, Association of Death Education and Counseling, the American Society for Reproductive Medicine, Postpartum Support International, Resolve, National Association of Social Workers, EMDRIA, and Florida Society for Clinical Hypnosis. Karyn served as treasurer, and past president of the Social Work/Mental Health Professional Council of Hadassah; and received the 2005 National Leadership Award, and past recipient of the Woman of Valor in 2004. Rosenberg is currently on the board of Professionals United for Parkland (PU4P) offering support and education for the community following the Marjorie Stoneman Douglas High School shooting. Rosenberg is a published contributing author in *The ABA Guide to Assisted Reproduction: Techniques, Legal Issues and Pathways to Success* (2016) and *Understanding the Journey: A Lifespan Approach to Working with Grieving People* (2019). She is currently on the strategic task force and has served on the board of trustees of her Synagogue, Temple Beth El-Boca Raton, and currently is part of the leadership council. Rosenberg is happily married to her husband, and raising two beautiful and smart daughters. When she isn't seeing clients, you will find her on her Peloton, reading a great book, or jamming out to live music.

Geoffrey Sher, MD, is the co-founder and executive medical director of Sher Institutes, is an internationally renowned expert in the field of Assisted

Reproductive Technology (ART), and has been influential in the births of more than 17,000 babies throughout his career. He is a pioneer in the field of Reproductive Immunology whose expertise is widely sought by patients from around the globe. He has treated patients from most of the fifty states and from more than twenty-five countries around the world. Sher trained under the "Father of IVF" Patrick Steptoe, and established the first private IVF program in the United States in 1982. Over the last forty-plus years, Sher and his medical teams have been on the leading edge of IVF research, pioneering significant breakthroughs that have become standard practice in the industry. He has hundreds of research studies, articles, and publications to his credit. Sher is still practicing in the field of reproductive medicine at the Sher Fertility Institute, New York, New York, and in Las Vegas, Nevada.

Kela Smith is a Holistic-Integrative Fertility and Hormone Doctor. She holds a PhD in Natural and Holistic Medicine as well as Double Board Certification as a Doctor of Natural Medicine (DNM) and Doctor of Humanitarian Medicine (DHM). Smith is also a Board-Certified Functional Nutritionist (BCFN) and a 5x Board-Certified Health Coach (BCHC). She founded The Hormone Puzzle Society and the Fertility Coach University. Smith has over twenty-five years of experience in integrative health and has published multiple books on fertility, hormones, and pregnancy as well as seven distinct online courses. She is also the host of The Hormone P.U.Z.Z.L.E Podcast, Solving-Infertility Summit, and Healthy Happy Pregnancy Summit.

Natasha Stamper, PharmD, is a clinical pharmacist and online fertility coach. She found her love for all things fertility while living in a remote Alaska village navigating her own IVF journey alone. After many miscarriages, two ectopic pregnancies, and one cervical ectopic she had her two miracle babies. Now with over twelve years of clinical pharmacy experience and her own experiences, she is so excited to be helping families all over the globe fulfill the dream of making their family complete. You can find her on Instagram at fertility_pharmacist or www.fertilitypharmacist.com.

Mark Surrey is the co-founder of Southern California Reproductive Center and a leader in the field of fertility and reproductive medicine, including reproductive surgery and in vitro fertilization (IVF). Surrey is a board-certified reproductive and endoscopic surgeon and serves as clinical professor in the Department of Obstetrics and Gynecology at the David Geffen School of Medicine at UCLA. He is also an associate director for advanced technologies at SCRC, providing IVF services to UCLA and Cedars-Sinai Medical Center. He has been in practice for more than twenty-five years. Surrey earned his bachelor's degree from the University of Pittsburgh and his MD from George Washington University. Following an internship and residency at UCLA Medical Center, he completed a research fellowship in reproductive endocrinology and an infertility fellowship at the University of London, Hammersmith Hospital. He then continued his training in preimplantation genetic diagnosis at the University of London and Monash University, Melbourne. A prolific researcher, Surrey has authored numerous publications for leading peer-reviewed journals including *Fertility and Sterility* and the *Journal of Assisted Reproduction and Genetics*. An active leader in this field, he is a former president of the American Association of Gynecologic Laparoscopists (AAGL), the largest association of minimally invasive gynecologists in the United States, and the leading organization of its kind worldwide. He is also a former president of the Pacific Coast Reproductive Society, the premier society of IVF specialists in the Western United States. Surrey continues to pursue the most advanced training in IVF, preimplantation genetic diagnosis (PGD), pelvic reconstructive surgery, microsurgery, and laparoscopic surgery, as one of the principal investigators of laparoscopic reconstructive surgery. Surrey has been voted one of the "Top 100 Health Professionals" and listed in "Best Doctors in America," and his expertise has also been featured nationally and internationally on media outlets including *The New York Times*, *The Los Angeles Times*, *Glamour*, *Parents*, CNN, Fox, CBS, ABC, NBC, among many others. Originally from Washington DC, Surrey now resides in Beverly Hills, with his wife and children.

Kendra A. Vargas, LCPC, PMH-C, is a culturally responsive and inclusive psychotherapist, clinical supervisor, consultant, and infertility trainer. She specializes in perinatal mental health and holds a Perinatal Mental Health Certificate through Postpartum Support International. Vargas is the founder of Authentically You Psychotherapy, a solo practice where she provides individual therapy and group therapy services. She has an ongoing Fertility Skills and Support Group for people utilizing Assisted Reproductive Technologies such as IUI and IVF, which is an area she has a deep, personal connection and compassion for.

Glossary of Terms and Abbreviations

Abnormal sperm parameters (ASP) abnormalities in a semen sample, such as a low sperm concentration or motility

Andrologist a professional that analyzes, washes, freezes, and thaws sperm

Anembryonic pregnancy a condition in early pregnancy in which implantation occurs but embryo development does not occur (also called a blighted ovum)

Aneuploid an embryo that has a high percentage of cells with the wrong amount of chromosomes

Anti-Mullerian hormone (AMH) a hormone commonly tested to estimate one's ovarian reserve

Anti-sperm antibodies (ASA) immune system proteins that can destroy sperm

Antral follicle count (AFC) the number of antral follicles present in one's ovaries obtained through the use of an ultrasound

Arrested (ARR) no longer showing signs of development

Artificial insemination (AI) insemination through a method other than ejaculation, including IUI

Assisted hatching (AH) mechanically creating a break in an embryo's shell (zona pellucida)

Assisted reproductive technologies (ART) medical procedures primarily used to address infertility which involve the manipulation of eggs, sperm, or embryos

Atretic (ATR) degenerate, often referring to eggs or embryos

Aunt Flo (AF) a common term for a period, which marks the beginning of a menstrual cycle

Azoospermia no sperm present in an ejaculate

Basal body temperature (BBT) your resting body temperature, which tends to increase following ovulation

Beta hCG blood test that measures the level of hCG in your blood to determine if embryo implantation occurred

Big fat negative (BFN) a negative pregnancy test

Big fat positive (BFP) a positive pregnancy test

Biopsy (BX) removing a sample of cells or tissue for laboratory testing or screening

Blastocoel the fluid-filled cavity which forms inside of an embryo at the blastocyst stage of development

Blastocyst (Blast or BL) a stage of embryo progression in which two distinct celllines and a cavity (blastocoel) form inside of an embryo

Body mass index (BMI) a measure of body fat based on one's height and weight

Cavitating the embryo is begun to form a cavity (blastocoel) and has entered the blastocyst stage of development

Chromosome long, wound strand of DNA; humans normally have twenty-three pairs in each of their cells

Cleavage stage an embryo consists of a few individual cells but has no yet compacted

Conventional insemination or IVF eggs and washed sperm are placed into a drop of media in hopes that fertilization will occur

Culture the media (fluid) embryos develop in

Cycle day (CD) refers to which day 1 is at during a menstrual cycle

Cryopreservation freezing eggs/embryos/sperm, usually through vitrification (flash freezing)

Cytomegalovirus (CMV) a common viral infection caused by a type of herpesvirus which can be transmitted to a fetus

Day 3 embryo transfer (D3 ET) an embryo transfer that occurs 3 days after insemination

Day 5 embryo transfer (D5 ET) an embryo transfer that occurs 5 days after insemination

Days post ovulation (DPO) the number of days that have passed since ovulation occurred

Days post transfer (DPT) the number of days that have passed since an embryo transfer occurred

Days post 5-day transfer (DP5DT) the number of days that have passed since a day 5 embryo transfer

Dilation and evacuation (D&E) a surgical procedure used to remove a fetus and all placental tissues after the first trimester of pregnancy

Diminished ovarian reserve (DOR) having fewer and lower-quality eggs in the ovaries compared to what is typically expected for individuals of the same age

Donor eggs eggs that were retrieved from a donor for use in IVF

Donor embryos embryos that were created through IVF and donated to another person or couple

Donor IVF (DIVF) IVF with the use of donor eggs

Early blastocyst (EB) an embryo's stage of development in which its cavity (blastocoel) consumes less than 50 percent of the embryo's space

Egg retrieval (ER) the process of removing eggs from their follicles in the ovaries for use in IVF. Also called an ovum pick up (OPU) or vaginal oocyte retrieval (VOR)

Embryo transfer (ET) the transfer of an embryo from a culture (petri) dish to the uterus

Embryologist professional that performs IVF (egg retrievals, insemination, embryo freezing/thawing, transfers, biopsies, etc.)

Empty Zona (EZ) see "fractured zona"

Endometriosis (Endo) the presence of endometrial-like tissue outside of the uterus

Estimated due date (EDD) the predicted date of delivery based on how advanced a pregnancy is

Estradiol (E2) a form of estrogen that is primarily produced by the ovaries that plays a crucial role in secondary sex characteristics, menstrual cycles, and fertility

Euploid an embryo with a high percentage of cells that contain the right amount of chromosomes

Expanded blastocyst (XB ot ExB) a stage of embryo development in which the shell (zona pellucida) surrounding the embryo begins to thin out as the embryo increases in size

Fetal heart rate (FHR) the rate at which a fetus's heart is beating

Follicle fluid-filled structure in which an egg resides within the ovaries

Follicle stimulating hormone (FSH) a hormone produced by the anterior pituitary gland of the brain which aids in sperm production and egg/follicle development

Follicular phase the phase between the start of the menstrual cycle and ovulation

Fractured zona (FZ) the shell surrounding an egg is fractured (broken). Also called an empty zona (EZ)

Fragmented an embryo that consists of cellular fragments (pieces of cells which broke off during development)

Freeze all (FA) cycle an IVF cycle in which all embryos that reach a certain stage of development are frozen, or cryopreserved, for future use. Also called a freeze-all blastocyst (FAB) cycle

Frozen embryo transfer (FET) an embryo is transferred to a uterus after being thawed from its frozen state

Gamete a sex cell (sperm or egg)

Germinal vesicle (GV) a very immature (early in development) egg

Gestational carrier (GC) someone who carries a pregnancy to term for intended parents

Gonadotropin releasing hormone(GnRH) a hormone produced by the hypothalamus in the brain which regulates sperm production in males and the menstrual cycle in females

GnRH Agonist a medication that initially promotes continuous FSH and LH production by the brain but then inhibits their production after a few days

GnRH Antagonist a medication that inhibits FSH and LH production by the brain to prevent ovulation from occurring

Haploid A cell that contains only one set of chromosomes, such as a mature egg or sperm cell

Hatched blastocyst (HB or HdB) an embryo which is completely hatched from its shell, or zona pellucida

Hatching blastocyst (HgB) an embryo that is hatching from its shell, or zona pellucida

Home pregnancy test (HPT) a pregnancy test that can be performed at home, usually with the use of urine

Hysterosalpingogram (HSG) a procedure in which contrast dye and an x-ray are used to observe the uterus and fallopian tubes

Hysteroscopy (Hyst) a procedure in which a small camera is inserted into the uterus to observe the uterine environment

In vitro fertilization (IVF) the process in which a sperm fertilizes an egg outside of the body

Immature egg an egg has not developed enough to be fertilized by a sperm, such as a germinal vesicle

Intracervical insemination (ICI) a sperm sample is injected into the cervix around the time of ovulation

Intracytoplasmic sperm injection (ICSI) one sperm is injected into a mature egg to hopefully achieve fertilization

Intrauterine insemination (IUI) a washed sperm sample is injected into the uterus around the time of ovulation

Known donor eggs (KDE) eggs that were retrieved from a donor whose identity is known to the intended parent(s)

Known donor embryo (KDE) embryos that were donated by a person/couple whose identity is known to the intended parent(s)

Known donor sperm (KDS) sperm that is from a donor whose identity is known to the intended parent(s)

Last menstrual period (LMP) the date that one's last menstrual cycle began

LH surge the rapid production of LH which triggers ovulation to occur

Luteal phase the time between ovulation and the subsequent menstrual cycle

Luteinizing hormone (LH) a hormone that is produced by the anterior pituitary gland which plays a role in testosterone production in males and egg maturation and ovulation in females

Male factor infertility (MFI) infertility as a result of male factors, such as a low sperm concentration or motility

Metaphase 1 (MI) an egg that has not completed its first meiotic division and is unable to be fertilized

Metaphase 2 (MII) an egg that has completed its first meiotic division and is able to be fertilized

Microscopic testicular sperm extraction (mTESE or microTESE) a specialized form of TESE during which providers use a microscope to examine the seminiferous tubules and extract those with high concentrations of sperm

Microsurgical epididymal sperm aspiration (MESA) sperm is aspirated from a small incision in the epididymis

Minimal stimulation ("mini stim") an IVF medication protocol in which a minimal amount of medications are administered to stimulate egg maturation

Miscarriage (MC) the unexpected ending of a pregnancy before twenty weeks of gestation

Missed miscarriage (MMC) a pregnancy is lost without awareness or symptoms of the loss

Morula (M or Mor), Latin for *mulberry* the stage of an embryo's development following the cleavage stage, in which the embryo's cells begin to condense

Mosaic an embryo that contains a mixture of cells with the correct and incorrect amount of DNA

Oligozoospermia low sperm count

Oligoasthenoteratozoospermia (OAT) low sperm count, motility, and morphology

Oocyte or ovum technical terms for an egg

Oral contraceptive pill (OCP) another term for a birth control pill

Ovarian hyperstimulation syndrome (OHSS) a condition in which the ovaries become overstimulated, typically from the administration of stimulation medications for IVF

Ovarian reserve the number and quality of eggs in one's ovaries

Ovulation the event which occurs near the middle of a menstrual cycle in which an egg is expelled from its follicle in the ovary

Ovulation induction (OI) a medical treatment that aims to improve ovulation patterns and fertility outcomes

Ovulation predictor kit (OPK) an over-the-counter kit that uses hormone levels inside of your body to predict when ovulation is approaching

Pelvic inflammatory disease (PID) an infection of the female reproductive tract that is usually caused by bacteria

Percutaneous epididymal sperm aspiration (PESA) sperm is aspirated from the epididymis through a small needle (no incision required)

Perivitelline space (PVS) the space between an egg's plasma membrane and its surrounding shell (zona pellucida)

Polycystic ovarian (ovary) syndrome (PCOS) a hormonal disorder that affects the ovaries in people during their childbearing years. PCOS is often associated with irregular menstrual cycles, excess androgen production, and polycystic ovaries

Pregnant until proven otherwise (PUPO) a common term used after an embryo transfer in which one is considered pregnant until a future pregnancy test confirms the pregnancy

Preimplantation genetic testing (PGT) a test that analyzes the DNA within the cell of an embryo

Preimplantation genetic testing for aneuploidy (PGT-A) a portion of an embryo's cells is analyzed to determine what percentage of the cells have the right amount of chromosomes

Preimplantation genetic testing for monogenic conditions (PGT-M) a portion of an embryo's cells is analyzed to determine if an embryo is affected by, a carrier of, or unaffected by a monogenic or single gene disorders

Preimplantation genetic testing for structural rearrangements (PGT-SR) a portion of an embryo's cells is screened for chromosomal imbalances resulting from parental structural rearrangements such as a translocations or inversions

Premature ovarian failure (POF): see
Premature ovarian failure (POF) see "primary ovarian insufficiency"

Primary infertility (PI) a person or couple has never been able to conceive a child

Primary ovarian insufficiency (POI) a condition in which the ovaries stop functioning normally before forty years of age

Products of conception (POC) a medical term used to describe any tissue derived from a pregnancy following an incomplete miscarriage, pregnancy termination, or delivery

Progesterone (P4) a hormone produced by the corpus luteum or placenta that plays a vital role in embryo implantation and pregnancy support

Progesterone in oil (PIO) an injectable form of progesterone that is dissolved in oil (usually sesame oil) and administered intramuscularly during the embryo transfer process

Prolactin a hormone produced by the brain primarily used for lactation; high levels can interfere with fertility in men and women

Pronucleus (PN) the structures found in a fertilized egg (zygote) that contain the genetic material from the egg and sperm and eventually fuse to form the nucleus of the embryo

Recurrent pregnancy loss (RPL) the occurrence of two or more consecutive pregnancy losses

Recurrent implantation failure (RIF) cases in which someone has had three failed embryo transfer attempts with good-quality embryos

Reproductive endocrinology and infertility (REI) a surgical subspecialty of obstetrics and gynecology that focuses on the treatment of infertility and hormonal dysfunctions related to reproduction in both males and females

Saline infusion sonogram (SIS) see "sonohysterogram"

Secondary infertility (SI) a person or couple who has already had a child experiences difficulty conceiving another child

Semen analysis (SA) analysis of a semen sample, particularly the sperm quality of the sample

Sexually transmitted infection (STI) infections spread mainly by contact with genitals or bodily fluids

Single mother by choice (SMBC) a woman (assigned female at birth) who is choosing to undergo fertility treatment without a partner

Sonohysterogram (SHG) diagnostic procedure, also referred to as a saline infusion sonogram, saline sonogram, or saline ultraouns, performed to evaluate the uterus using saline

Spontaneous abortion (SAB) see "miscarriage"

Stimulation (stim) the process of administering medications that stimulate follicles to grow and eggs to mature

Teratozoospermia a high number of abnormal looking sperm in a semen sample

Testicular sperm aspiration (TESA): sperm are aspirated from the testes through a small needle (no incision required)

Testicular sperm extraction (TESE) a small piece of the seminiferous tubules are surgically removed and the sperm inside of them are extracted

Therapeutic donor insemination (TDI) the use of donor sperm for the purpose of artificial insemination. Also known as artificial insemination by donor

Thyroid stimulating hormone (TSH) a hormone produced by the pituitary gland that plays a role in regulating thyroid function and metabolism

Timed intercourse (TIC) intercourse that occurs around the time of ovulation

Transvaginal ultrasound (TVUS) a internal ultrasound of the pelvic area in which the image is projected through a probe (transducer) that is inserted into the vagina

Trigger warning (TW) the following content may cause you emotional pain or trigger certain emotions

Trying to conceive (TTC) attempting to conceive a pregnancy

Two-week wait (TWW) the time between ovulation or an embryo transfer until a pregnancy test can be taken

Ultrasound (US) a procedure in which internal organs are examined using a probe (transducer)

Unfertilized oocyte (0PN) an egg that does not show signs of fertilization following insemination

White blood cell (WBC) blood cells that primarily serve to fight infections

Zona pellucida (ZP) the glycoprotein layer (shell) that surrounds and protects an egg and early embryo.

Zygote (2PN) a fertilized egg (one cell)

0PN an unfertilized egg with no pronuclei present

1PN embryo with 1 pronucleus following insemination

2PN (zygote) embryo with 2 pronuclei following insemination

3PN embryo with 3 pronuclei following insemination

Notes

Preface

1. Definition of Infertility: A Committee Opinion (2023). https://www.asrm.org/practice-guidance/practice-committee-documents/denitions-of-infertility/. Accessed September 17, 2024.

Chapter 2

1. Shridharani, Anand, Ryan C. Owen, Osama O. Elkelany, and Edward D. Kim. "The Significance of Clinical Practice Guidelines on Adult Varicocele Detection and Management." *Asian Journal of Andrology* 18, no. 2 (2016): 269–75. https://doi.org/10.4103/1008-682X.172641.

Chapter 7

1. "What Is Assisted Reproductive Technology? | Reproductive Health | CDC." May 14, 2024. https://www.cdc.gov/art/whatis.html.
2. Das, Mausumi, and Weon-Young Son. "In Vitro Maturation (IVM) of Human Immature Oocytes: Is It Still Relevant?" *Reproductive Biology and Endocrinology : RB&E* 21 (2023). https://doi.org/10.1186/s12958-023-01162-x.
3. Sahay, Dr. Richika. "Top 10 Reasons for Slow Growing Follicles in IVF Which No One Will Tell You." *India IVF*, November 3, 2023. https://www.indiaivf.in/blog/top-reasons-slow-follicles-ivf/.
4. Lele, Prasad R., N. Nagaraja, Yoginder Singh, and Barun Kumar Chakraborty. "Characteristics of Empty Follicular Syndrome during In Vitro Fertilization Embryo Transfer and Its Association with Various Etiologies in Comparatively Young Patients." *Journal of Human Reproductive Sciences* 13, no. 1 (2020): 51–5. https://doi.org/10.4103/jhrs.JHRS_96_19.
5. Fleming, Steven, David Morroll, and Martine Nijs. "Sperm Separation and Selection Techniques to Mitigate Sperm DNA Damage." *Life* 15, no. 2 (February 14, 2025): 302. https://doi.org/10.3390/life15020302.

6   Legacy. "Posthumous Sperm Retrieval." December 10, 2022. https://www.givelegacy.com/resources/posthumous-sperm-retrieval/.

7   Jellerette-Nolan, Teru, Amber R. Cooper, Kevin J. Doody, John E. Nichols, John K. Park, Robin L. Poe-Zeigler, Andrew F. Khair, Laura M. Stong, Richard J. Paulson, and Gaurang S. Daftary. "Real-World Experience with Intravaginal Culture Using INVOCELL: An Alternative Model for Infertility Treatment." *F&S Reports* 2, no. 1 (March 1, 2021): 9–15. https://doi.org/10.1016/j.xfre.2020.11.003.

8   "Intracytoplasmic Sperm Injection (ICSI) for Non–Male Factor Indications: A Committee Opinion (2020)." https://www.asrm.org/practice-guidance/practice-committee-documents/intracytoplasmic-sperm-injection-icsi-for-nonmale-factor-indications-a-committee-opinion-2020/. Accessed September 18, 2024.

9   Lacamara, Celeste, Carolina Ortega, Sonia Villa, Ricardo Pommer, and Juan Enrique Schwarze. "Are Children Born from Singleton Pregnancies Conceived by ICSI at Increased Risk for Congenital Malformations When Compared to Children Conceived? A Systematic Review and Meta-Analysis." *JBRA Assisted Reproduction* 21, no. 3 (2017): 251–9. https://doi.org/10.5935/1518–0557.20170047.

10 Klonoff-Cohen, Hillary, and Mounika Polavarapu. "Assessing the Relationship Between Traditional In Vitro Fertilization and Birth Defects: A Systematic Review and Meta-Analysis." *Journal of IVF-Worldwide* 1, no. 4 (December 18, 2023). https://doi.org/10.46989/001c.91039.

11 Ruan, Jing Ling, Shan Shan Liang, Jia Ping Pan, Zhi Qin Chen, and Xiao Ming Teng. "Artificial Oocyte Activation with Ca2+ Ionophore Improves Reproductive Outcomes in Patients with Fertilization Failure and Poor Embryo Development in Previous ICSI Cycles." *Frontiers in Endocrinology* 14 (August 11, 2023). https://doi.org/10.3389/fendo.2023.1244507.

12 Nicholson, C.L., M. Dean, A. Attia, P.A. Milne, and S. Martins da Silva. "Artificial Oocyte Activation Improves ICSI Outcomes Following Unexplained Fertilization Abnormalities." *Reproductive BioMedicine Online*, June 21, 2024. https://www.rbmojournal.com/article/S1472-6483(24)00516-9/fulltext.

13 Glatthorn, Haley N., and Alan Decherney. "The Efficacy of Add-Ons: Selected IVF 'Add-on' Procedures and Future Directions." *Journal of Assisted Reproduction and Genetics* 39, no. 3 (March 2022): 581–9. https://doi.org/10.1007/s10815-022-02410-6.

14 Kahyaoglu, Inci, Berfu Demir, Ayten Turkkanı, Ozgur Cınar, Serdar Dilbaz, Berna Dilbaz, and Leyla Mollamahmutoglu. "Total Fertilization Failure: Is It the End of the Story?" *Journal of Assisted Reproduction and Genetics* 31, no. 9 (September 2014): 1155–60. https://doi.org/10.1007/s10815-014-0281-5.

15 Batha, Sara, Goli Ardestani, Olcay Ocali, Pam Jarmuz, Denis A. Vaughan, C. Brent Barrett, and Denny Sakkas. "Day after Rescue ICSI: Eliminating Total Fertilization Failure after Conventional IVF with High Live Birth Rates Following Cryopreserved Blastocyst Transfer." *Human Reproduction* 38, no. 7 (July 5, 2023): 1277–83. https://doi.org/10.1093/humrep/dead097.

16 Zhu, Xiaxuan, Tian Tian, Dina Jiesisibieke, Shilin Fang, Nan Zhang, Jinxi Ma, Yuqi Xia, et al. "Clinical Outcome of Different Embryo Transfer Strategies after Late Rescue ICSI Procedure: A 10-Year Total Fertilisation Failure Cohort Study." *BMC*

Pregnancy and Childbirth 23, no. 1 (July 31, 2023): 549. https://doi.org/10.1186/s12884-023-05859-0.

17. Du, Tong, Yun Wang, Yong Fan, Shiyi Zhang, Zhiguang Yan, Weina Yu, Qianwen Xi, et al. "Fertility and Neonatal Outcomes of Embryos Achieving Blastulation on Day 7: Are They of Clinical Value?" *Human Reproduction* 33, no. 6 (June 1, 2018): 1038–51. https://doi.org/10.1093/humrep/dey092.

18. Yin, Beining, Sichen Li, Lin Sun, Zhiyi Yao, Yueyue Cui, Congli Zhang, and Yile Zhang. "Comparing Day 5 versus Day 6 Euploid Blastocyst in Frozen Embryo Transfer and Developing a Predictive Model for Optimizing Outcomes: A Retrospective Cohort Study." *Frontiers in Endocrinology* 14 (January 4, 2024): 1302194. https://doi.org/10.3389/fendo.2023.1302194.

19. Brolinson, Marja, Xiaohong Liu, Molly Bergen, Samad Jahandideh, Kathleen Devine, Micah J. Hill, Alan H. DeCherney, Phillip A. Romanski, and Benjamin S. Harris. "What is The Reproductive Potential of Euploid Day-6 and Day-7 Blastocysts Compared to Euploid Day-5 Blastocysts?" *Fertility and Sterility*, 79th Scientific Congress of the American Society for Reproductive Medicine 120, no. 4, Supplement (October 1, 2023): e65. https://doi.org/10.1016/j.fertnstert.2023.08.737.

20. Hu, Juwei, Juan Zheng, Jie Li, Haiyue Shi, Hua Wang, Bangxu Zheng, Kun Liang, Chunhao Rong, and Liming Zhou. "D6 High-Quality Expanded Blastocysts and D5 Expanded Blastocysts Have Similar Pregnancy and Perinatal Outcomes Following Single Frozen Blastocyst Transfer." *Frontiers in Endocrinology* 14 (November 9, 2023): 1216910. https://doi.org/10.3389/fendo.2023.1216910.

21. Embryoman. "Embryo Arrest." *Remembryo*, February 8, 2019. https://www.remembryo.com/embryo-arrest/.

22. Yang, Yang, Liyang Shi, Xiuling Fu, Gang Ma, Zhongzhou Yang, Yuhao Li, Yibin Zhou, et al. "Metabolic and Epigenetic Dysfunctions Underlie the Arrest of in Vitro Fertilized Human Embryos in a Senescent-like State." *PLOS Biology* 20, no. 6 (June 30, 2022): e3001682. https://doi.org/10.1371/journal.pbio.3001682.

23. Racowsky, Catherine, Judy E. Stern, William E. Gibbons, Barry Behr, Kimball O. Pomeroy, and John D. Biggers. "National Collection of Embryo Morphology Data into Society for Assisted Reproductive Technology Clinic Outcomes Reporting System: Associations among Day 3 Cell Number, Fragmentation and Blastomere Asymmetry, and Live Birth Rate." *Fertility and Sterility* 95, no. 6 (May 1, 2011): 1985–9. https://doi.org/10.1016/j.fertnstert.2011.02.009.

24. Grysole, Camille, Simon Phillips, Lise Preaubert, and Louise Lapensée. "What Are the Chances of Success for Couples Performing an IVF Cycle with Only Poor Quality Day-3 Embryos Cultured to the Blastocyst Stage?" *Fertility and Sterility*, 2019 ASRM Abstract Issue 112, no. 3, Supplement (September 1, 2019): e160. https://doi.org/10.1016/j.fertnstert.2019.07.535.

25. Zou, Haowen, James M. Kemper, Elizabeth R. Hammond, Fengqin Xu, Gensheng Liu, Lintao Xue, Xiaohong Bai, et al. "Blastocyst Quality and Reproductive and Perinatal Outcomes: A Multinational Multicentre Observational Study." *Human Reproduction (Oxford, England)* 38, no. 12 (October 24, 2023): 2391–9. https://doi.org/10.1093/humrep/dead212.

26. Zhao, Yan-Yu, Yang Yu, and Xiao-Wei Zhang. "Overall Blastocyst Quality, Trophectoderm Grade, and Inner Cell Mass Grade Predict Pregnancy Outcome in Euploid Blastocyst Transfer Cycles." *Chinese Medical Journal* 131, no. 11 (June 5, 2018): 1261–7. https://doi.org/10.4103/0366-6999.232808.

27. Kirillova, Anastasia, Sergey Lysenkov, Maria Farmakovskaya, Yulia Kiseleva, Bella Martazanova, Nona Mishieva, Aydar Abubakirov, and Gennady Sukhikh. "Should We Transfer Poor Quality Embryos?" *Fertility Research and Practice* 6, no. 1 (February 19, 2020): 2. https://doi.org/10.1186/s40738-020-00072-5.

28. Maheshwari, Abha, Vasha Bari, Jennifer L Bell, Siladitya Bhattacharya, Priya Bhide, Ursula Bowler, Daniel Brison, et al. "Transfer of Thawed Frozen Embryo versus Fresh Embryo to Improve the Healthy Baby Rate in Women Undergoing IVF: The E-Freeze RCT." *Health Technology Assessment (Winchester, England)* 26, no. 25 (May 2022): 1–142. https://doi.org/10.3310/AEFU1104.

29. Wang, Ange, Anthony Santistevan, Karen Hunter Cohn, Alan Copperman, John Nulsen, Brad T. Miller, Eric Widra, Lynn M. Westphal, and Piraye Yurttas Beim. "Freeze-Only versus Fresh Embryo Transfer in a Multicenter Matched Cohort Study: Contribution of Progesterone and Maternal Age to Success Rates." *Fertility and Sterility* 108, no. 2 (August 1, 2017): 254–261.e4. https://doi.org/10.1016/j.fertnstert.2017.05.007.

30. Maheshwari, Abha, Vasha Bari, Jennifer L. Bell, Siladitya Bhattacharya, Priya Bhide, Ursula Bowler, Daniel Brison, et al. "Transfer of Thawed Frozen Embryo versus Fresh Embryo to Improve the Healthy Baby Rate in Women Undergoing IVF: The E-Freeze RCT." *Health Technology Assessment (Winchester, England)* 26, no. 25 (May 2022): 1–142. https://doi.org/10.3310/AEFU1104.

31. Stormlund, Sacha, Negjyp Sopa, Anne Zedeler, Jeanette Bogstad, Lisbeth Prætorius, Henriette Svarre Nielsen, Margaretha Laczna Kitlinski, et al. "Freeze-All versus Fresh Blastocyst Transfer Strategy during in Vitro Fertilisation in Women with Regular Menstrual Cycles: Multicentre Randomised Controlled Trial." *BMJ (Clinical Research Ed.)* 370 (August 5, 2020): m2519. https://doi.org/10.1136/bmj.m2519.

32. Weiss, Marissa Steinberg, Chongliang Luo, Yujia Zhang, Yong Chen, Dmitry M. Kissin, Glen A. Satten, and Kurt T. Barnhart. "Fresh vs. Frozen Embryo Transfer: New Approach to Minimize the Limitations of Using National Surveillance Data for Clinical Research." *Fertility and Sterility* 119, no. 2 (February 1, 2023): 186–94. https://doi.org/10.1016/j.fertnstert.2022.10.021.

33. Garbhini, Putu Githa, Anom Suardika, A.A.N. Anantasika, I.B. Putra Adnyana, I. Made Darmayasa, Nono Tondohusodo, and Jaqueline Sudiman. "Day-3 vs. Day-5 Fresh Embryo." *JBRA Assisted Reproduction* 27, no. 2 (2023): 163–8. https://doi.org/10.5935/1518-0557.20220027.

34. Rao, Jinpeng, Feng Qiu, Shen Tian, Ya Yu, Ying Zhang, Zheng Gu, Yiting Cai, Fan Jin, and Min Jin. "Clinical Outcomes for Day 3 Double Cleavage-Stage Embryo Transfers versus Day 5 or 6 Single Blastocyst Transfer in Frozen–Thawed Cycles: A Retrospective Comparative Analysis." *Journal of International Medical Research* 49, no. 12 (December 2021): 030006052110624. https://doi.org/10.1177/03000605211062461.

35 Wang, Ningling, Xinxi Zhao, Meng Ma, Qianqian Zhu, and Yao Wang. "Effect of Day 3 and Day 5/6 Embryo Quality on the Reproductive Outcomes in the Single Vitrified Embryo Transfer Cycles." *Frontiers in Endocrinology* 12 (April 23, 2021). https://doi.org/10.3389/fendo.2021.641623.

36 Agha-Hosseini, Marzieh, Leila Hashemi, Ashraf Aleyasin, Marzieh Ghasemi, Fatemeh Sarvi, Maryam Shabani Nashtaei, and Mahshad Khodarahmian. "Natural Cycle versus Artificial Cycle in Frozen-Thawed Embryo Transfer: A Randomized Prospective Trial." *Turkish Journal of Obstetrics and Gynecology* 15, no. 1 (March 2018): 12–17. https://doi.org/10.4274/tjod.47855.

37 Wang, A., J. Kort, and L.M. Westphal. "Medicated versus Natural Frozen Embryo Transfer for Euploid Embryos." *Fertility and Sterility*, Scientific Congress Supplement: Oral and Poster Session Abstracts 110, no. 4, Supplement (September 1, 2018): e402. https://doi.org/10.1016/j.fertnstert.2018.07.1154.

38 Carosso, Andrea Roberto, Nicole Brunod, Claudia Filippini, Alberto Revelli, Bernadette Evangelisti, Stefano Cosma, Fulvio Borella, Stefano Canosa, Chiara Benedetto, and Gianluca Gennarelli. "Reproductive and Obstetric Outcomes Following a Natural Cycle vs. Artificial Endometrial Preparation for Frozen–Thawed Embryo Transfer: A Retrospective Cohort Study." *Journal of Clinical Medicine* 12, no. 12 (June 13, 2023): 4032. https://doi.org/10.3390/jcm12124032.

39 "Role of Assisted Hatching in in Vitro Fertilization: A Guideline (2022)." https://www.asrm.org/practice-guidance/practice-committee-documents/the-role-of-assisted-hatching-in-in-vitro-fertilization-a-guideline-2022/. Accessed September 26, 2024.

40 Child, Tim J., Aysha Bevan, Rebecca Frettsome-Hook, Jo Craig, Sevanna Shahbazian, and Ginny Mounce. "A Randomised Controlled Blinded Trial Assessing the Effectiveness of Embryoglue as an Embryo Transfer Medium in IVF Cycles." *Fertility and Sterility*, 77th Scientific Congress of the American Society for Reproductive Medicine 116, no. 3, Supplement (September 1, 2021): e4. https://doi.org/10.1016/j.fertnstert.2021.07.019.

41 Heymann, Devorah, Liat Vidal, Yuval Or, and Zeev Shoham. "Hyaluronic Acid in Embryo Transfer Media for Assisted Reproductive Technologies." *The Cochrane Database of Systematic Reviews* 2020, no. 9 (September 2, 2020): CD007421. https://doi.org/10.1002/14651858.CD007421.pub4.

42 Zhang, Hui xia, Fei Li, Haixia Jin, Wen yan Song, Yingchun Su, and Gang Li. "Effect of Retained Embryos on Pregnancy Outcomes of in Vitro Fertilization: A Matched Retrospective Cohort Study." *BMC Pregnancy and Childbirth* 23 (January 4, 2023): 5. https://doi.org/10.1186/s12884-022-05315-5.

43 Roberts, Alexis-Danielle, Richard Schmidt, and Meera Shah. "Split Happens: A Case of Consecutive Monozygotic Twin Pregnancies Following Elective Single-Embryo Transfer in a 40-Year Old Woman Using Donor Oocytes." *Journal of Assisted Reproduction and Genetics* 35, no. 8 (August 2018): 1529–32. https://doi.org/10.1007/s10815-018-1218-1.

44 MacKenna, A., J.E. Schwarze, J. Crosby, and F. Zegers-Hochschild. "Factors Associated with Embryo Splitting and Clinical Outcome of Monozygotic Twins in Pregnancies after IVF and ICSI." *Human Reproduction Open* 2020, no. 1 (May 15, 2020): hoaa024. https://doi.org/10.1093/hropen/hoaa024.

45 "Guidance on the Limits to the Number of Embryos to Transfer: A Committee Opinion (2021)." https://www.asrm.org/practice-guidance/practice-committee-documents/guidance-on-the-limits-to-the-number-of-embryos-to-transfer-a---committee-opinion-2021/. Accessed September 26, 2024.

46 "Multifetal Pregnancy Reduction." https://www.acog.org/clinical/clinical-guidance/committee-opinion/articles/2017/09/multifetal-pregnancy-reduction. Accessed September 26, 2024.

47 Wong, Kai Mee, Sebastiaan Mastenbroek, and Sjoerd Repping. "Cryopreservation of Human Embryos and Its Contribution to in Vitro Fertilization Success Rates." *Fertility and Sterility* 102, no. 1 (July 1, 2014): 19–26. https://doi.org/10.1016/j.fertnstert.2014.05.027.

48 Cimadomo, Danilo, Antonio Capalbo, Paolo Emanuele Levi-Setti, Daria Soscia, Giovanna Orlando, Elena Albani, Valentina Parini, et al. "Associations of Blastocyst Features, Trophectoderm Biopsy and Other Laboratory Practice with Post-Warming Behavior and Implantation." *Human Reproduction* 33, no. 11 (November 1, 2018): 1992–2001. https://doi.org/10.1093/humrep/dey291.

49 Shu, Yimin, Jill Watt, Janice Gebhardt, Jennifer Dasig, Julie Appling, and Barry Behr. "The Value of Fast Blastocoele Re-Expansion in the Selection of a Viable Thawed Blastocyst for Transfer." *Fertility and Sterility* 91, no. 2 (February 1, 2009): 401–6. https://doi.org/10.1016/j.fertnstert.2007.11.083.

50 Allen, Meagan, Lyndon Hale, Daniel Lantsberg, Violet Kieu, John Stevens, Catharyn Stern, David K. Gardner, and Yossi Mizrachi. "Post-Warming Embryo Morphology Is Associated with Live Birth: A Cohort Study of Single Vitrified-Warmed Blastocyst Transfer Cycles." *Journal of Assisted Reproduction and Genetics* 39, no. 2 (February 1, 2022): 417–25. https://doi.org/10.1007/s10815-021-02390-z.

51 FertilitySmarts. "Embryo Freezing and Thawing: What You Need to Know." February 27, 2019. https://www.fertilitysmarts.com/embryo-freezing-and-thawing-what-you-need-to-know/.

Chapter 8

1 Franasiak, Jason M., Eric J. Forman, Kathleen H. Hong, Marie D. Werner, Kathleen M. Upham, Nathan R. Treff, and Richard T. Scott. "The Nature of Aneuploidy with Increasing Age of the Female Partner: A Review of 15,169 Consecutive Trophectoderm Biopsies Evaluated with Comprehensive Chromosomal Screening." *Fertility and Sterility* 101, no. 3 (March 2014): 656–63.e1. https://doi.org/10.1016/j.fertnstert.2013.11.004.

2 Picchetta, Ludovica, Christian S. Ottolini, Helen C. O'Neill, and Antonio Capalbo. "Investigating the Significance of Segmental Aneuploidy Findings in Preimplantation Embryos." *F&S Science* 4, no. 2 (May 2023): 17–26. https://doi.org/10.1016/j.xfss.2023.03.004.

3 Girardi, Laura, Munevver Serdarogullari, Cristina Patassini, Maurizio Poli, Marco Fabiani, Silvia Caroselli, Onder Coban, et al. "Incidence, Origin, and Predictive

Model for the Detection and Clinical Management of Segmental Aneuploidies in Human Embryos." *American Journal of Human Genetics* 106, no. 4 (April 2, 2020): 525–34. https://doi.org/10.1016/j.ajhg.2020.03.005.

4   Babariya, D., E. Fragouli, S. Alfarawati, K. Spath, and D. Wells. "The Incidence and Origin of Segmental Aneuploidy in Human Oocytes and Preimplantation Embryos." *Human Reproduction (Oxford, England)* 32, no. 12 (December 1, 2017): 2549–60. https://doi.org/10.1093/humrep/dex324.

5   Kubicek, David, Miroslav Hornak, Jakub Horak, Rostislav Navratil, Gabriela Tauwinklova, Jiri Rubes, and Katerina Vesela. "Incidence and Origin of Meiotic Whole and Segmental Chromosomal Aneuploidies Detected by Karyomapping." *Reproductive Biomedicine Online* 38, no. 3 (March 2019): 330–9. https://doi.org/10.1016/j.rbmo.2018.11.023.

6   Lin, Joanna, Wendy Vitek, and Erin L. Scott. "Order from Chaos: A Case Report of a Healthy Live Birth from a Genetically 'Chaotic' Embryo." *F&S Reports* 3, no. 4 (December 2022): 301–4. https://doi.org/10.1016/j.xfre.2022.10.003.

7   Zhang, Ying Xin, Jang Jih Chen, Sunanta Nabu, Queenie Sum Yee Yeung, Ying Li, Jia Hui Tan, Wanwisa Suksalak, et al. "The Pregnancy Outcome of Mosaic Embryo Transfer: A Prospective Multicenter Study and Meta-Analysis." *Genes* 11, no. 9 (August 21, 2020): 973. https://doi.org/10.3390/genes11090973.

8   Capalbo, Antonio, Maurizio Poli, Laura Rienzi, Laura Girardi, Cristina Patassini, Marco Fabiani, Danilo Cimadomo, et al. "Mosaic Human Preimplantation Embryos and Their Developmental Potential in a Prospective, Non-Selection Clinical Trial." *American Journal of Human Genetics* 108, no. 12 (December 2, 2021): 2238–47. https://doi.org/10.1016/j.ajhg.2021.11.002.

9   Viotti, Manuel, Andrea R. Victor, Frank L. Barnes, Christo G. Zouves, Andria G. Besser, James A. Grifo, En-Hui Cheng, et al. "Using Outcome Data from One Thousand Mosaic Embryo Transfers to Formulate an Embryo Ranking System for Clinical Use." *Fertility and Sterility* 115, no. 5 (May 2021): 1212–24. https://doi.org/10.1016/j.fertnstert.2020.11.041.

10 Capalbo, Antonio, Maurizio Poli, Laura Rienzi, Laura Girardi, Cristina Patassini, Marco Fabiani, Danilo Cimadomo, et al. "Mosaic Human Preimplantation Embryos and Their Developmental Potential in a Prospective, Non-Selection Clinical Trial." *American Journal of Human Genetics* 108, no. 12 (December 2, 2021): 2238–47. https://doi.org/10.1016/j.ajhg.2021.11.002.

11 Viotti, Manuel, Andrea R. Victor, Frank L. Barnes, Christo G. Zouves, Andria G. Besser, James A. Grifo, En-Hui Cheng, et al. "Using Outcome Data from One Thousand Mosaic Embryo Transfers to Formulate an Embryo Ranking System for Clinical Use." *Fertility and Sterility* 115, no. 5 (May 2021): 1212–24. https://doi.org/10.1016/j.fertnstert.2020.11.041.

12 Viotti, Manuel, Ermanno Greco, James A. Grifo, Mitko Madjunkov, Clifford Librach, Murat Cetinkaya, Semra Kahraman, et al. "Chromosomal, Gestational, and Neonatal Outcomes of Embryos Classified as a Mosaic by Preimplantation Genetic Testing for Aneuploidy." *Fertility and Sterility* 120, no. 5 (November 2023): 957–66. https://doi.org/10.1016/j.fertnstert.2023.07.022.

13 Neal, Shelby A., L. Sun, C. Jalas, S.J. Morin, T.A. Molinaro, and R.T. Scott. "When Next-Generation Sequencing-Based Preimplantation Genetic Testing for Aneuploidy (PGT-A) Yields an Inconclusive Report: Diagnostic Results and Clinical Outcomes after Re Biopsy." *Journal of Assisted Reproduction and Genetics* 36, no. 10 (October 2019): 2103–9. https://doi.org/10.1007/s10815-019-01550-6.

14 Treff, Nathan R., and Diego Marin. "The 'Mosaic' Embryo: Misconceptions and Misinterpretations in Preimplantation Genetic Testing for Aneuploidy." *Fertility and Sterility* 116, no. 5 (November 2021): 1205–11. https://doi.org/10.1016/j.fertnstert.2021.06.027.

15 Capalbo, Antonio, Maurizio Poli, Laura Rienzi, Laura Girardi, Cristina Patassini, Marco Fabiani, Danilo Cimadomo, et al. "Mosaic Human Preimplantation Embryos and Their Developmental Potential in a Prospective, Non-Selection Clinical Trial." *American Journal of Human Genetics* 108, no. 12 (December 2, 2021): 2238–47. https://doi.org/10.1016/j.ajhg.2021.11.002.

16 Reignier, Arnaud, Jenna Lammers, Paul Barriere, and Thomas Freour. "Can Time-Lapse Parameters Predict Embryo Ploidy? A Systematic Review." *Reproductive Biomedicine Online* 36, no. 4 (April 2018): 380–7. https://doi.org/10.1016/j.rbmo.2018.01.001.

17 Navratil, Rostislav, Jakub Horak, Miroslav Hornak, David Kubicek, Maria Balcova, Gabriela Tauwinklova, Pavel Travnik, and Katerina Vesela. "Concordance of Various Chromosomal Errors among Different Parts of the Embryo and the Value of Re-Biopsy in Embryos with Segmental Aneuploidies." *Molecular Human Reproduction* 26, no. 4 (April 24, 2020): 269–76. https://doi.org/10.1093/molehr/gaaa012.

18 Victor, Andrea R., Darren K. Griffin, Alan J. Brake, Jack C. Tyndall, Alex E. Murphy, Laura T. Lepkowsky, Archana Lal, et al. "Assessment of Aneuploidy Concordance between Clinical Trophectoderm Biopsy and Blastocyst." *Human Reproduction (Oxford, England)* 34, no. 1 (January 1, 2019): 181–92. https://doi.org/10.1093/humrep/dey327.

19 Grkovic, Steve, Maria V. Traversa, Mark Livingstone, and Steven J. McArthur. "Clinical Re-Biopsy of Segmental Gains—the Primary Source of Preimplantation Genetic Testing False Positives." *Journal of Assisted Reproduction and Genetics* 39, no. 6 (June 2022): 1313–22. https://doi.org/10.1007/s10815-022-02487-z.

20 Lin, Joanna, Wendy Vitek, and Erin L. Scott. "Order from Chaos: A Case Report of a Healthy Live Birth from a Genetically 'Chaotic' Embryo." *F&S Reports* 3, no. 4 (December 2022): 301–4. https://doi.org/10.1016/j.xfre.2022.10.003.

21 Franasiak, Jason M., Eric J. Forman, Kathleen H. Hong, Marie D. Werner, Kathleen M. Upham, Nathan R. Treff, and Richard T. Scott. "The Nature of Aneuploidy with Increasing Age of the Female Partner: A Review of 15,169 Consecutive Trophectoderm Biopsies Evaluated with Comprehensive Chromosomal Screening." *Fertility and Sterility* 101, no. 3 (March 2014): 656–63.e1. https://doi.org/10.1016/j.fertnstert.2013.11.004.

22 Kubicek, David, Miroslav Hornak, Jakub Horak, Rostislav Navratil, Gabriela Tauwinklova, Jiri Rubes, and Katerina Vesela. "Incidence and Origin of Meiotic Whole and Segmental Chromosomal Aneuploidies Detected by Karyomapping."

Reproductive Biomedicine Online 38, no. 3 (March 2019): 330–9. https://doi.org/10.1016/j.rbmo.2018.11.023.

23. Bardos, Jonah, Jaclyn Kwal, Wayne Caswell, Samad Jahandideh, Melissa Stratton, Michael Tucker, Alan DeCherney, Kate Devine, Micah Hill, and Jeanne E. O'Brien. "Reproductive Genetics Laboratory May Impact Euploid Blastocyst and Live Birth Rates: A Comparison of 4 National Laboratories' PGT-A Results from Vitrified Donor Oocytes." *Fertility and Sterility* 119, no. 1 (January 2023): 29–35. https://doi.org/10.1016/j.fertnstert.2022.10.010.

Chapter 11

1. Chavarro, J.E., J.W. Rich-Edwards, B. Rosner, and W.C. Willett. "A Prospective Study of Dairy Foods Intake and Anovulatory Infertility." *Human Reproduction (Oxford, England)* 22, no. 5 (May 2007): 1340–7. https://doi.org/10.1093/humrep/dem019.
2. Group, Environmental Working. "Dirty Dozen™ Fruits and Vegetables with the Most Pesticides." https://www.ewg.org/foodnews/dirty-dozen.php. Accessed September 26, 2024.
3. Group, Environmental Working. "Clean Fifteen™ Conventional Produce with the Least Pesticides." https://www.ewg.org/foodnews/clean-fifteen.php. Accessed September 26, 2024.
4. Zhu, Lei, Bin Zhou, Xi Zhu, Feng Cheng, Ying Pan, Yi Zhou, Yong Wu, and Qingna Xu. "Association Between Body Mass Index and Female Infertility in the United States: Data from National Health and Nutrition Examination Survey 2013-2018." *International Journal of General Medicine* 15 (February 19, 2022): 1821–31. https://doi.org/10.2147/IJGM.S349874.
5. Pandey, Shilpi, Suruchi Pandey, Abha Maheshwari, and Siladitya Bhattacharya. "The Impact of Female Obesity on the Outcome of Fertility Treatment." *Journal of Human Reproductive Sciences* 3, no. 2 (2010): 62–7. https://doi.org/10.4103/0974-1208.69332.
6. Mann, Uday, Benjamin Shiff, and Premal Patel. "Reasons for Worldwide Decline in Male Fertility." *Current Opinion in Urology* 30, no. 3 (May 2020): 296–301. https://doi.org/10.1097/MOU.0000000000000745.
7. Ricci, E., S. Al-Beitawi, S. Cipriani, A. Alteri, F. Chiaffarino, M. Candiani, S. Gerli, P. Viganó, and F. Parazzini. "Dietary Habits and Semen Parameters: A Systematic Narrative Review." *Andrology* 6, no. 1 (January 2018): 104–16. https://doi.org/10.1111/andr.12452.
8. Afeiche, Myriam C., Audrey J. Gaskins, Paige L. Williams, Thomas L. Toth, Diane L. Wright, Cigdem Tanrikut, Russ Hauser, and Jorge E. Chavarro. "Processed Meat Intake Is Unfavorably and Fish Intake Favorably Associated with Semen Quality Indicators among Men Attending a Fertility Clinic." *The Journal of Nutrition* 144, no. 7 (July 2014): 1091–8. https://doi.org/10.3945/jn.113.190173.

9   Chavarro, Jorge E., Lidia Mínguez-Alarcón, Jaime Mendiola, Ana Cutillas-Tolín, José J. López-Espín, and Alberto M. Torres-Cantero. "Trans Fatty Acid Intake Is Inversely Related to Total Sperm Count in Young Healthy Men." *Human Reproduction (Oxford, England)* 29, no. 3 (March 2014): 429–40. https://doi.org/10.1093/humrep/det464.

11 Rozati, Roya, P.P. Reddy, P. Reddanna, and Rubina Mujtaba. "Role of Environmental Estrogens in the Deterioration of Male Factor Fertility." *Fertility and Sterility* 78, no. 6 (December 2002): 1187–94. https://doi.org/10.1016/s0015-0282(02)04389-3.

12 Afeiche, M., P.L. Williams, J. Mendiola, A.J. Gaskins, N. Jørgensen, S.H. Swan, and J.E. Chavarro. "Dairy Food Intake in Relation to Semen Quality and Reproductive Hormone Levels among Physically Active Young Men." *Human Reproduction (Oxford, England)* 28, no. 8 (August 2013): 2265–75. https://doi.org/10.1093/humrep/det133.

13 Robbins, Wendie A., Lin Xun, Leah Z. FitzGerald, Samantha Esguerra, Susanne M. Henning, and Catherine L. Carpenter. "Walnuts Improve Semen Quality in Men Consuming a Western-Style Diet: Randomized Control Dietary Intervention Trial." *Biology of Reproduction* 87, no. 4 (October 2012): 101. https://doi.org/10.1095/biolreprod.112.101634.

15 Ricci, Elena, Paola Viganò, Sonia Cipriani,Edgardo Somigliana, Francesca Chiaffarino, Alessandro Bulfoni, and Fabio Parazzini. "Coffee and Caffeine Intake and Male Infertility: A Systematic Review." *Nutrition Journal* 16 (June 24,2017): 37. https://doi.org/10.1186/s12937-017-0257-2.

16 Nguyen-Thanh, Tung, Ai-Phuong Hoang-Thi, and Dang Thi Anh Thu. "Investigating the Association between Alcohol Intake and Male Reproductive Function: A Current Meta-Analysis." *Heliyon* 9, no. 5 (May 1, 2023): e15723. https://doi.org/10.1016/j.heliyon.2023.e15723.

18 Dai, Jing-Bo, Zhao-Xia Wang, and Zhong-Dong Qiao. "The Hazardous Effects of Tobacco Smoking on Male Fertility." *Asian Journal of Andrology* 17, no. 6 (2015): 954–60. https://doi.org/10.4103/1008-682X.150847.

21 CDC. "About Lead and Other Heavy Metals and Reproductive Health." *Reproductive Health and the Workplace*, April 22, 2024. https://www.cdc.gov/niosh/reproductive-health/prevention/lead-metals.html.

22 Bloom, Michael S., Patrick J. Parsons, Amy J. Steuerwald, Enrique F. Schisterman, Richard W. Browne, Keewan Kim, Gregory A. Coccaro, Giulia C. Conti, Natasha Narayan, and Victor Y. Fujimoto. "Toxic Trace Metals and Human Oocytes during in Vitro Fertilization (IVF)." *Reproductive Toxicology (Elmsford, N.Y.)* 29, no. 3 (June 2010): 298–305. https://doi.org/10.1016/j.reprotox.2010.01.003.

23 Bloom, Michael S., Victor Y. Fujimoto, Amy J. Steuerwald, Gloria Cheng, Richard W. Browne, and Patrick J. Parsons. "Background Exposure to Toxic Metals in Women Adversely Influences Pregnancy during in Vitro Fertilization (IVF)." *Reproductive Toxicology (Elmsford, N.Y.)* 34, no. 3 (November 2012): 471–81. https://doi.org/10.1016/j.reprotox.2012.06.002.

24 Manouchehri, Aliasghar, Samira Shokri, Mohadeseh Pirhadi, Mohammad Karimi, Saber Abbaszadeh, Ghazal Mirzaei, and Mahmoud Bahmani. "The Effects of Toxic Heavy Metals Lead, Cadmium and Copper on the Epidemiology of Male and

Female Infertility." *JBRA Assisted Reproduction* 26, no. 4 (2022): 627–30. https://doi.org/10.5935/1518-0557.20220013.

25 Kumar, Sunil. "Occupational and Environmental Exposure to Lead and Reproductive Health Impairment: An Overview." *Indian Journal of Occupational and Environmental Medicine* 22, no. 3 (2018): 128–37. https://doi.org/10.4103/ijoem.IJOEM_126_18.

27 Jeong, Kyoung Sook, Hyewon Park, Eunhee Ha, Jiyoung Shin, Yun-Chul Hong, Mina Ha, Hyesook Park, et al. "High Maternal Blood Mercury Level Is Associated with Low Verbal IQ in Children." *Journal of Korean Medical Science* 32, no. 7 (July 2017): 1097–104. https://doi.org/10.3346/jkms.2017.32.7.1097.

28 Jeong, Kyoung Sook, Hyewon Park, Eunhee Ha, Jiyoung Shin, Yun-Chul Hong, Mina Ha, Hyesook Park, et al. "High Maternal Blood Mercury Level Is Associated with Low Verbal IQ in Children." *Journal of Korean Medical Science* 32, no. 7 (July 2017): 1097–104. https://doi.org/10.3346/jkms.2017.32.7.1097.

29 Henriques, Magda Carvalho, Susana Loureiro, Margarida Fardilha, and Maria Teresa Herdeiro. "Exposure to Mercury and Human Reproductive Health: A Systematic Review." *Reproductive Toxicology* 85 (April 1, 2019): 93–103. https://doi.org/10.1016/j.reprotox.2019.02.012.

30 Kumar, Sunil, and Anupama Sharma. "Cadmium Toxicity: Effects on Human Reproduction and Fertility." *Reviews on Environmental Health* 34, no. 4 (December 18, 2019): 327–38. https://doi.org/10.1515/reveh-2019-0016.

31 Qu, Jingwen, Qiang Wang, Xiaomei Sun, and Yongjun Li. "The Environment and Female Reproduction: Potential Mechanism of Cadmium Poisoning to the Growth and Development of Ovarian Follicle." Ecotoxicology and Environmental Safety 244 (October 1, 2022): 114029. https://doi.org/10.1016/j.ecoenv.2022.114029.

32 Wieczorek, Katarzyna, Dorota Szczęsna, Michał Radwan, Paweł Radwan, Kinga Polańska, Anna Kilanowicz, and Joanna Jurewicz. "Exposure to Air Pollution and Ovarian Reserve Parameters." *Scientific Reports* 14, no. 1 (January 3, 2024): 461. https://doi.org/10.1038/s41598-023-50753-6.

33 Pizzorno, Joseph. "Environmental Toxins and Infertility." *Integrative Medicine: A Clinician's Journal* 17, no. 2 (April 2018): 8–11. https://www.ncbi.nlm.nih.gov/pmc/articles/PMC6396757/.

34 Jangid, Pooja, Umesh Rai, Radhey Shyam Sharma, and Rajeev Singh. "The Role of Non-Ionizing Electromagnetic Radiation on Female Fertility: A Review." *International Journal of Environmental Health Research* 33, no. 4 (April 2023): 358–73. https://doi.org/10.1080/09603123.2022.2030676.

35 Negi, Pooja, and Rajeev Singh. "Association between Reproductive Health and Nonionizing Radiation Exposure." *Electromagnetic Biology and Medicine* 40, no. 1 (January 2, 2021): 92–102. https://doi.org/10.1080/15368378.2021.1874973.

Index

Note: Page numbers in *italics* refer to tables and figures.

0PN (0 pronuclei) 98
1PN (1 pronucleus) 98
2PN (2 pronuclei) 98
3PN (3 pronuclei) 99

acceptance 182
acrosome 15
adenomyosis 39, 155
adhesion 29, 33
adoption 228, 232–3
   emotional aspects 230–1
   level of openness 229
   types 228
adrenal disorders 36–7
advancing age 40
air pollution 203–4
alloimmune implantation
       dysfunction 160–2
alloimmune recognition 163
alpha-adrenergic agonists 19
American Society for Reproductive
       Medicine (ASRM) viii, 123
ampulla 28, 29
anatomy
   female reproductive system *28*
      cervix 29
      fallopian tubes (oviducts) 28–9
      ovaries 27
      uterus 29
      vagina 29
   male reproductive system *14*
      organs and structures 13–14
      physiology 14–15
      sperm *15*, 15–16

androgen 35, 36
andropause 21. *See also* late onset
       hypogonadism
androstenedione 37
anembryonic pregnancy (blighted
       ovum) 150
aneuploid 130, 135, 138, 142, 154
anger 183
anovulation 34
anti-Müllerian hormone (AMH) 40, 52
antiovarian antibodies (autoimmune
       oophoritis) 166
antiphospholipid antibodies
       (APAs) 164–5
antiphospholipid syndrome (APS)
       165
antisperm antibodies (ASAs) 23–4
antithyroid antibodies (ATA) 166
antral follicle count (AFC) 40, 55, 70
apposition 33
aromatase inhibitors 66
artificial oocyte activation (AOA) 97
Asherman's syndrome 38, 155
assisted hatching (AH) 117, 123
assisted reproductive technologies
       (ART) 77
autoantibodies 164
   antiovarian antibodies (AOA) 166
   antiphospholipid antibodies
       (APAs) 164–5
   antithyroid antibodies (ATA) 166
autoimmune disorders 37
autoimmune implantation
       dysfunction 164–6

autoimmune thyroid disease (AITD)   166
autosomes   135
azoospermia   viii, 17

bargaining   183
basal body temperature (BBT)   31, 62
belly breathing   185
bicornuate uterus   38
biochemical (chemical) pregnancy   33, 150
birth control pills   71–2
Bisphenol A (BPA)   193, 197, 200
blastocoel   109
blastocyst   32
  embryo grading   110–11, *113*
blastomere   32, 100, 106
block to polyspermy   16
body mass index (BMI)   195
boundaries   182
box breathing   183–4
breathing exercises   184
bromocriptine   66

cabergoline   66
capacitation   15, 32
Center for Disease Control (CDC)   77
cervical agenesis   158
cervix   29
chaotic embryo   139, 147
Child Welfare Information Gateway   228
chlamydia screening   23, 60
choline   196
chromosome   111, 135, 136
cleavage-stage embryos. *See* day 3 embryo grading
clomiphene citrate (Clomid)   65
Coenzyme Q10 (CoQ10)   196, 199
compassionate transfer   131
complete molar pregnancy   151
complex aneuploid   139
complex carbohydrates   194, 198–9
conception   15, 32, 62
congenital adrenal hyperplasia (CAH)   36
corpus luteum   31, 33

corticosteroids (prednisone and dexamethasone)   167
couples therapy   187
cryoprotectant agents (CPAs)   126
cryotank (Dewar)   127
cryptorchidism   20
cumulus cells   81
Cushing's syndrome   36
cystic fibrosis   59
cytotoxic T cells   162

DABDA   181
day 3 embryo grading   106–8, 112
dehydroepiandrosterone (DHEA)   37
denial   183
density gradient centrifugation (DGC)   90
denudation   82
depression   183
Dialectical Behavior Therapy (DBT)   182
diminished ovarian reserve (DOR)   40, 52, 54, 87, 215
DNA fragmentation index (DFI)   23
domestic infant adoption
  benefits   231
  challenges   232
  emotional aspects   230–1
  expert guidance   233
  level of openness   233
  paths and options   228–9
  phases   229–30
donor eggs   215
  adoption ineligibility   223
  considerations   219
  donation ineligibility   217
  identification   218–19
  process   216–17
  reasons for conception   215–16
  reasons for donation   216
  receiving process   217–18
  splitting up eggs   218
donor embryos   220
  adoption process   223
  dividing embryo sets   222
  information about adopted embryos   221

known vs. anonymous
  donations 221–2
 process 220–1
 reasons to use 222
donor sperm 208–10
 choosing and receiving 212–13
 considerations for use 213–14
 safety of sperm banks 210–11
Down Syndrome 142
DQ alpha/HLA genetic matching 164
 partial DQ alpha genetic
  matching 164
 total (complete) alloimmune genetic
  matching 164

early pregnancy loss (EPL, miscarriage,
  spontaneous abortion) 150
ectopic pregnancy 151
egg freezing (oocyte
  cryopreservation) 88–9
egg maturity 83–5
egg quality 42, 99, 105
egg retrieval (ovum pickup, OPU)
 in IVF lab 81–3
 preparation 79
 procedure 78
 procedure setup 79–81
egg stripping/denudation 82
egg thawing (oocyte warming) 88–9
ejaculatory duct 14
embryo arrest 104–6
embryo biopsy 124, 135
embryo development 100, 101–3,
  104
embryo disposition 130–1
embryo freezing (vitrification or flash
  freezing) 37, 40, 126–8
EmbryoGlue® 117
embryo grading 106
 and success rates 111
embryo incompetence 150, 155–6
embryo rebiopsy 145
embryo splitting 121–3, 122
embryo thawing (warming) 129–30
embryo transfers 111–12
 after transfer 120–1
 blastocyst 113
 day 3 112

fresh 111
frozen 111
medicated (programmed,
  artificial) 113–15
multiple embryo transfer 121,
  123
preparation 117
procedure 117–18
unmedicated (natural) 115
empty follicles 87–8
empty follicle syndrome (EFS) 87
endocrine disrupting chemicals
  (EDCs) 200
endometrial biopsy 58
endometrial polyps 155
endometrioma 39
endometriosis 39, 165
endometritis 38
endometrium 29, 151, 157
environmental hazards 160
epididymis 13
erectile dysfunction (ED) 20–1. See
  also impotence
estradiol (E2) 27, 54
estrogen 69
estrogen priming 72
euploid 138
expanded blastocyst 110

fallopian tubes (oviducts) 28–9, 39–40
FDA 196, 210, 211, 216, 220
female factor infertility (FFI) 33–4, 43
fertility medications 65–6
 considerations 73
 side effects 71
fertility specialist 45
 appointment 46–8
 considerations 45–6
 consultation 49
 initial consultation 48–9
 receiving diagnosis and treatment
  plan 49
fertilization 96–100
fibroids 38
fimbriae 28, 31
flare protocol 72
folate 198
follicle 78, 80

follicle-stimulating hormone (FSH) 15, 31, 35, 53, 54
Fragile X syndrome 37
Free T3 (FT3) 53
Free T4 (FT4) 53
fresh embryo transfers 69, 112
frozen embryo transfers (FETs) 69, 104, 111–12

Gardner scale 109
gene 135
genetic carrier screening 59–60, 211, 221
genetic conditions 19, 21–2, 59, 211
genetic counseling 22
genetic testing facility 125
genomic activation 104
germinal vesicles (GVs) 84
Girardi, Laura 147
Gonadotropin-releasing hormone (GnRH) 34
　agonists 67–8
　antagonists 68
gonadotropins 66, 67
gonorrhea screening 60
Grave's disease 36
grief and loss 171
　coping with 182–6
　external factors 179–80
　pregnancy-related losses 174
　primary and secondary loss 181
　relating to family planning 174–8
　seeking help 186–8
group therapy 187

Hashimoto's thyroiditis 36
healthy fats 194, 197
heavy metals 201
　cadmium 202
　lead 201–2
　mercury 202
hormone replacement therapy 37
human chorionic gonadotropin (hCG) 33, 66, 68, 121
human leukocyte antigen (HLA) system 163
hyaluronan-enriched transfer medium (HETM) 117

hyaluronidase 15, 82
hydrosalpinx 40, 57
hyperprolactinemia 36
hyperthyroidism 36, 159
hypogonadism 19–20
hypothalamic amenorrhea 34–5
hypothalamic-pituitary-adrenal (HPA) axis 37
hypothyroidism 36, 166
hysterosalpingo-contrast sonography (HyCoSy) 56–7
hysterosalpingography (HSG) 39, 57, 58
hysteroscopy 57

immunity screening 53
immunologic implantation dysfunction (IID) 150, 155, 160–1, 164
　classes 161–6
　treatment options 167
implantation 33
impotence 20
individual therapy 187
infectious disease screening 52–3, 210
infertility viii, ix, 41. See also fertility specialist
　causes 51–2
　defined vii
　diagnostic procedures
　　chlamydia and gonorrhea screening 60
　　endometrial biopsy 58
　　fertility assessment scan (FAS) or pelvic exam 55
　　genetic carrier screening 59–60
　　hysterosalpingo-contrast sonography (HyCoSy) 56–7
　　hysterosalpingography (HSG) 57
　　hysteroscopy 57
　　karyotypes 60
　　laparoscopy and dye test 57
　　saline infusion sonogram (SIS) 55–6
　　semen analysis/seminal fluid analysis (SFA) 59
　　sonohysterogram (SHG) 55–6

gestures and actions that
    hurt   235–8
  support strategies   238–9
  treatment options   61–2
    intrauterine insemination
      (IUI)   63–4
    natural cycle tracking and timed
      intercourse   62–3
    ovulation induction (OI)   63
    in vitro fertilization (IVF)   64
infertility counselor   9, 10
infertility trauma   1
  causes   1–3
  effect on relationships with
    others   8–9
  effect on relationships with
    partners   6–8
  emotions   3–4
  resources   9–10
  self-esteem   4–5
  symptoms   4
infundibulum   28
inner cell mass (ICM)   109, 123
insemination   93
  conventional IVF insemination
    (IVF)   94
  intracytoplasmic sperm injection
    (ICSI)   94–6
insulin resistance   35
Interstate Compact on the Placement
  of Children (ICPC)   230
intracervical insemination (ICI)   63–4
intracytoplasmic sperm injection
  (ICSI)   17–19, 22, 23, 82–3,
  87, 94–6, 100
intralipid (IL) infusion   162, 164, 166
intralipid (IL) therapy   167
intrauterine growth restriction
  (IUGR)   165
intrauterine insemination (IUI)   17, 19,
  21, 24, 56, 63–7, 90
intravaginal culture (IVC)   94
intravenous immunoglobulin-G (IVIG)
  therapy   167
invasion   33, 151
in vitro fertilization (IVF)   vii, 2, 17, 19,
  22, 37, 40, 54, 66, 77, 132,
  215, 224

egg freezing   88–9
egg maturation process   86–7
egg maturity   83–5
empty follicles   87
freezing sperm   92–3
medications   66–7
  classes   67–9
  minimal stimulation   69–70
  monitoring   70–1
  ovum pick up (OPU) (see egg
    retrieval)
  sperm collection   89
  sperm information   89
  sperm preparation   90–2
  thawing   88–9
in vitro maturation (IVM)   85–6
isthmus   29

journaling   5, 183

karyotype   60
Klinefelter syndrome   18
Kubler Model   183
Kübler-Ross, Elisabeth   183

laparoscopy   57
late onset hypogonadism   21
late pregnancy loss (LPL)   151
lifestyle factors   20, 41, 160
low-fat dairy products   193
Lupron   67
Luteal phase defect (LPD)   35
luteinizing hormone (LH)   15, 31,
  53–4, 62
Lymphocyte Immunization Therapy
  (LIT)   167

M1 oocyte   83, 84
M2 oocyte   83
male factor infertility (MFI)   16, 24
  andropause   21
  azoospermia   17
  cryptorchidism   20
  disorders and abnormalities   17–22
  erectile dysfunction (ED)   20–1
  hypogonadism   19–20
  oligoasthenoteratospermia
    (OAT)   18–19

oligospermia 17–18
  retrograde ejaculation 19
  teratospermia
    (teratozoospermia) 18
  varicocele 17
maternal-to-zygotic transition
  (MZT) 104, 121
medicated FET cycles 114
medication management 188
meiosis 83
memorial service 183
menstrual cycle 30
  follicular phase 31
  luteal phase 31–2
  menstrual phase 30–1
  ovulation 31
metformin 66
microdissection testicular sperm
  extraction (micro-TESE) 17, 90
microsurgical epididymal sperm
  aspiration (MESA) 89
minimal stimulation 69–70
missed (silent) miscarriage 150
mittelschmerz 62
molar pregnancy (hydatidiform
  mole) 151
monosomy 138
mosaicism/mosaic 139, 141, 144–5
mullerian agenesis (MRKH
  syndrome) 38
Müllerian anomalies 38, 158
Müllerian ducts 158
multifetal pregnancy reduction 124
multiple sclerosis 19
myometrium 29
National Institute of Child Health and
  Human Development 196
National Society of Genetic
  Counselors 148
natural cycle tracking 62, 113
natural killer (NK) cells 162
Next Generation Sequencing
  (NGS) 140, 142
non-ionizing radiation 203
non-obstructive azoospermia 17

obstructive azoospermia 17
oligoasthenoteratospermia (OAT) 18–19
oligo-ovulation 34
oligospermia 17–18
omega-3 fatty acids 194, 198
oocyte activation 32, 96
operating room (OR) 79
oral contraceptive pills (OCP, both
  control pills) 115
orchiopexy 20
ovarian hyperstimulation syndrome
  (OHSS) 68, 71, 86
ovarian reserve 40
ovaries 27
ovulation 31, 34, 62, 65, 115
ovulation induction (OI) 63
ovulation predictor kits (OPKs) 62
ovulatory dysfunction 34, 37

partial molar pregnancy 151
pelvic exam (fertility assessment
  scan) 55
pelvic inflammatory disease (PID) 60
penis 19
per- and polyfluoroalkyl substances
  (PFAS) 200–1
percutaneous epididymal sperm
  aspiration (PESA) 89
perimetrium 29
Perinatal Mental Health Certification
  (PMH-C) 187
pesticides 193, 202
phthalates 201
physiological intracytoplasmic sperm
  injection (PICSI) 97
placebo pills 72
placenta 33, 115, 121, 151
plant-based protein sources 194
polar body 83, 95
polycystic ovary syndrome
  (PCOS) 34, 53, 66
polypectomy 38, 155
polyspermy 96
poor-quality embryos 111, 125, 153–4
posthumous sperm retrieval (PSR) 93
Postpartum Support International
  (PSI) 186, 187

pregnancy loss   150–4, 178
preimplantation genetic testing
    (PGT)   125–6, 130, 135–7
  and embryo transfer status   140
  normal versus abnormal
    results   140–1
preimplantation genetic testing for
    aneuploidy (PGT-A)   135,
    146, 156
  accuracy   143–4
  considerations   146–7
  embryo re-biopsy   144–5
  mosaic embryos   141–2
  reasons to perform   142–3
  results   138–40
preimplantation genetic testing for
    monogenic conditions
    (PGT-M)   60, 137
preimplantation genetic testing for
    structural rearrangements
    (PGT-SR)   60, 135
premature ovarian failure   37
premenstrual syndrome (PMS)   32
primary hypogonadism   19
primary ovarian insufficiency (POI)   37,
    52, 53
progesterone (P4)   27, 35, 68–9, 114,
    115
progesterone deficiency   155
prolactin   54, 66
prostate gland   14

radiation   18, 203–4
Radical Acceptance   182
reactive oxygen species (ROS)   106,
    192
recurrent early pregnancy loss   150
recurrent pregnancy loss (RPL)
    152–3, 165
reproductive failure   150, 170
  causes   153–4
reproductive health   191
  environmental toxins   200
  factors influencing   191–2
  female fertility optimization   192–6
  male fertility optimization   197–9
reproductive hormone testing   53–4
rescue ICSI   100

retrograde ejaculation   19
ribonucleic acid (RNA)   105

saline infusion sonogram
    (sonohysterogram, SHG)   55–6
scrotum   13, 20, 89
secondary hypogonadism   19
seed and soil concept   149
segmental aneuploidies   138–9, 147,
    148
selective estrogen receptor modulators
    (SERMs)   20
semen   15, 22
  analysis results
    antisperm antibodies
      (ASAs)   23–4
    sperm DNA fragmentation
      (SDF)   23
    sperm morphology   22
    sperm motility   22
    total sperm count   22
seminal fluid analysis (SFA)   59
seminal vesicle   14
septate uterus   158
Sertoli cells   15
sexually transmitted infections
    (STIs)   57, 159
single gene condition   137
spermatogenesis   15
spermatozoa (sperm)   15–16, 89
  anatomy   16
  concentration   22
  cryopreservation   21
  donation   208–9
  freezing (cryopreservation)   21
  morphology   18, 22
  motility   22, 198
  preparation methods   90–2
  production   15, 17, 18, 20
  separation devices   91
sperm DNA fragmentation (SDF)   23,
    92
sporadic (not recurrent) EPL   150, 156
stillbirth   151
structural abnormalities
  fallopian tubes   39–40
  uterus   38–9
submucosal fibroids   155

surrogacy 224
   considerations 226–7
   coping 226
   reasons 224–5
swim-up method 91, *92*
syphilis 53

teratospermia (teratozoospermia) 18
testes (testicles) 13
testicular sperm aspiration (TESA) 89
testicular sperm extraction (TESE) 17, 89
testosterone 15, 54
testosterone replacement therapy (TRT) 19, 21
TH-1 cytokines 162, 167
TH-2 cytokines 162
thin endometrium 158–9
third-party (or donor-assisted) reproduction 205
   reasons to consider 205–6
   time to consider 206
   triggering emotions 207
thrombophilia 165
thyroid hormone supplementation 36
thyroid hormone testing 53
thyroid peroxidase antibodies (TPO-Ab) 53
thyroid stimulating hormone (TSH) 53
timed intercourse (TIC) 62, 63, 65, 66
transabdominal ultrasound 55
transvaginal ultrasound 63
transvaginal ultrasound scan (TVUS) 55
trial transfers 118
triggers 180

triploidy 97
trisomy 138
Trisomy 21 (Down syndrome) 40
trophectoderm epithelium (TE) 109
two-week wait (TWW) 177
type 2 diabetes 35

ultra-processed trans-fats 193
unexplained infertility 41, 164
unicornuate uterus 38
urethra 14
uterine adhesions 38
uterine congenital abnormalities 38, 156
uterine fibroids (leiomyomas) 38, 155
uterine lesions 154–5
uterine polyps 38
uterine scar tissue 38, 39
uterus 29, 38–9
uterus didelphys 38

vagina 29
vaginal oocyte retrieval (VOR) 78
vanishing twin syndrome 124
Varicella 53
varicocele 17, 18
vas deferens 14
vitamin D deficiency 196
vitrification device 127
volatile organic compounds (VOCs) 106
vulva 29

World Health Organization (WHO) vii

zygote 100